The Physiology of
CESTODES

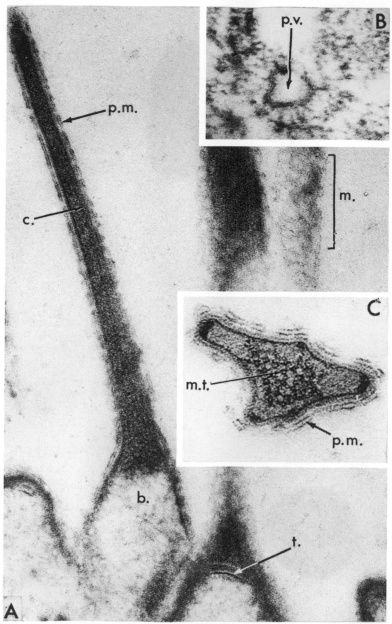

(*Frontispiece*) Ultrastructure of the tegument of *Echinococcus granulosus*. A. Vertical section of a microthrix (× 88,000). B. Vesicle (pinocytotic?) in distral cytoplasm (× 118,000). C. Cross-section of a microthrix (× 163,000). b. base; c. electron dense core; m. 'mosaic' pattern seen in tangential section; m.t. microtubule; p.m. plasma membrane; p.v. pinocytotic vesicle?; t. tube-like structure. For further interpretation, see Fig. 5.] (After Jha & Smyth, 1969.)

The Physiology of
CESTODES

J. D. SMYTH
Professor of Zoology
Australian National University
Canberra

W. H. FREEMAN AND COMPANY
SAN FRANCISCO

UNIVERSITY REVIEWS IN BIOLOGY

General Editor: J. E. TREHERNE

Advisory Editors: Sir VINCENT WIGGLESWORTH, F.R.S.
M. J. WELLS
T. WEIS-FOGH

Printed in the United States of America.
Library of Congress Catalog Card Number: 71-98694
Standard Book Number: 7167 0676-8

Published in Great Britain by Oliver & Boyd, Ltd.,
Edinburgh and London.

Preface

The aim of this book, which is a companion volume to *The Physiology of Trematodes* (Oliver & Boyd, 1966), is to give an account of the physiology of cestodes from the egg, through the larval stages, to the adult worm.

No account of the physiology of this group has hitherto been published. This is, perhaps, not surprising, for only within recent years has the application of biochemical, biophysical, physiological and immunological techniques enabled anything approaching an integrated account of the physiology of this group to emerge. In the past, cestode species of medical or veterinary interest have probably received an undue share of the attention of biologists. This has undoubtedly resulted in exclusion of other species, which, although not of economic importance, may in fact be more suitable for work of an experimental nature.

Since physiological studies of any group of organisms nowadays involve investigations at molecular, cellular, tissue, organ, whole organism and ecological levels, it is clear that questions, fundamental to whole areas of biology—such as morphogenesis—must inevitably be raised in a text of this nature.

An attempt has been made here to survey the literature in the major languages, up to about mid-1967. The author is acutely conscious, however, of the rate at which biological concepts are changing and of the mass of material being published at the time this volume is going to press.

One of the major difficulties in writing a modern scientific text is to decide what to leave out; and the content of any book inevitably reflects, to some degree, the interests—and limitations—of the writer. The areas covered in this text are those in which fundamental advances appear to have been made in the last decade, advances which have thrown light on the basic understanding of parasitism as a phenomenon. Time alone will show how relevant has been the final choice of topics to the way in which this field ultimately develops.

J. D. SMYTH

Acknowledgements

I am grateful to the following, who have read and commented critically on various sections of this text: Dr C. Bryant, Dr J. A. Clegg, Mr D. Heath, Dr M. J. Howell, Dr P. Janssens, Dr R. K. Jha, Dr N. Tate, Dr J. C. Pearson, Dr H. Smith, Mrs J. M. Shield, Mrs M. M. Smyth and Dr L. T. Threadgold. Mr Heath and Mrs Shield have generously allowed me to make use of unpublished material.

The text figures have been contributed by Mrs H. Miller, Mrs A. Warrener and my wife, to whom my thanks are due. Mrs Miller was largely responsible for the final form of the illustrations and for much detailed checking of the manuscript, and I am grateful for the care and patience with which she carried out this task. Most of the illustrations have been redrawn from original sources to conform to a uniform style and acknowledgement is made to numerous authors, editors and publishers in this respect.

I am indebted to the following publishers and editors for permission to use materials: Academic Press Inc.; *Acta Parasitologica Polonica*; Allen Press; American Physiological Socicty; Blackwell Scientific Publications; Cambridge University Press; *Canadian Journal of Zoology*; Commonwealth Agricultural Bureaux; English Universities Press, Ltd.; *Endeavour*; Iowa Academy of Science; *Journal of Parasitology*; Lancaster Press; Masson et Cie; Macmillan (Journals), Ltd.; New York Academy of Sciences; Pergamon Press, Ltd.; Polish Scientific Press; W. B. Saunders & Co.; Springer-Verlag; Verlag für Recht & Gesellschaft, A. G.; World Health Organization.

The typing of the manuscript was entirely the work of Mrs R. Rawlinson and I am indebted to her patience and skill in the setting out and preparation of this text.

Contents

To the Student

The Scope of this Book

It is now recognised that in the study of a group of the animal kingdom, it is important to be able to present an ' integrated ' account of the group in terms of modern biology. Thus, the morphologist cannot ignore the physiology of the organisms. Similarly, the biochemist, the physiologist and the electron microscopist must view their results in relation to structure and behaviour. In the case of a parasitic group, a further factor—the relationship between host and parasite—must be taken into account.

Although this book deals with cestodes, it is now evident that these organisms can serve as models for the study of basic biological problems, and they are so regarded in this text.

Suggested Approach to Reading

In considering the physiology it is assumed that the reader is familiar with the basic morphology of a cestode, but attention is drawn in Chapter 2, to those features, especially the tegument, which are of particular physiological interest. Chapter 3 deals with the physiology of the vertebrate alimentary canal, a knowledge of which is fundamental to the understanding of the biology of the adult cestode. The biochemistry and metabolism of the group are dealt with in Chapters 4–6, but for a proper understanding of these areas some knowledge of morphology is essential. Chapters 7–9 deal with the morphogenesis of cestodes from egg to adult and the physiological aspects of the life cycle; these chapters can be read without any knowledge of the previous chapters. Similarly, Chapter 10, which deals with the problems of *in vitro* culture, can be read as a separate entity, but a general knowledge of the biology of a cestode is assumed.

The final Chapters (11–13) deal with the relationship between a parasite and its host; a problem which leads into the study of immunology, a field now recognised as one of the most fundamental in cell biology. As this topic is of increasing importance to parasitologists, and is one about which it is rather difficult to obtain information except from medically orientated textbooks, the basic concepts of immunity have been dealt with in some detail.

The Physiology of
CESTODES

1: The Cestodes:
General Considerations

General Account

The Cestodes represent a group of organisms which present many features of exceptional physiological interest. They are, for example, almost unique amongst parasites in that the adult occupies only one particular type of habitat—the alimentary canal—in one particular group of animals, the vertebrates. Moreover, the known exceptions to this generalisation occur in sites related to the intestine, such as the bile duct, gall bladder or pancreatic ducts so that the biotope is essentially confined to the alimentary canal or its derivatives.

The only adult forms which occur in hosts other than vertebrates are members of the sub-class Cestodaria, whose physiology is entirely unknown, and a few neotenic (p. 132) forms in oligochaetes.

The dominating morphological features of adult cestodes are (a) an elongated, tape-like body—a form elegantly adapted to its tubular environment, and (b) the absence of an alimentary canal either in adult or larval stages. The latter feature is of considerable physiological importance, for clearly the external surface of the body must thus serve not only as a protective covering but also as a metabolically active layer through which secretions can be transported, nutritive material absorbed, and waste material eliminated.

Ultrastructure studies, discussed later (p. 7), show that the external body-covering consists of what is virtually a ' naked ' cytoplasmic layer i.e. one unprotected by a resistant cuticle. Such a surface would (theoretically) be strongly antigenic in a host tissue site, a supposition which is borne out by immunological studies. In contrast with the adult, larval cestodes can occur in almost any organ of both vertebrate and invertebrate hosts, although most larvae show a predilection for a particular site. In tissue sites, an analogy has been drawn[400-402] between cysticerci and the embryos of the placental mammals, with regard to their relationship with the host tissue (Fig. 53).

During recent years it has become clear that one of the most important—yet least studied—areas in cestode physiology is that of the morphology, cytology, ultrastructure and metabolic activities of the host and parasite tissues at their immediate border of contact, i.e. the *host-parasite interface*. It has generally been assumed that since cestodes are primarily lumen-inhabiting forms they absorb the digested, or partly-digested, material available in the gut lumen or that available from the neighbourhood of the mucosa—a region which has been termed the *paramucosa*[296]. There is now convincing evidence that in species in which the scolex becomes deeply embedded in the intestinal mucosa (e.g. *Echinococcus granulosus*, p. 182), the scolex behaves essentially as a tissue parasite and the free strobilar region as a lumen-dwelling one. In some species at least, then, the scolex region of a worm appears to be capable of absorbing some materials *directly* (?) from the intestinal wall[430] although the strobilar part of the worm is (presumably) absorbing from the contents of the intestinal lumen. The physiological problems arising from this complex situation are discussed later (pp. 34, 90).

Problems of the Life Cycle

With rare exceptions (e.g. *Hymenolepis nana*), cyclophyllidean cestodes require at least one intermediate host, and pseudophyllidean cestodes two (or more rarely three) intermediate hosts. Although the life cycles of the other classes of cestodes (such as Trypanorhyncha) have been worked out, their physiology has been almost entirely neglected. Thus, the physiological problems of the life cycle have been studied mainly in the Cyclophyllidea and the Pseudophyllidea, classes in which experimental material is readily available.

In this volume, an attempt is made to examine the physiology of the egg, larval and adult stages of cestodes, and, in particular, to analyse those factors which may influence or determine the development of the various stages in the cestode life cycle.

The study in depth of the physiology of an organism must nowadays necessarily involve investigations at the molecular, cellular, tissue, organ, the whole organism and ecological levels. Only when such studies have been made, is it possible to obtain an integrated picture of the physiology. Such studies raise questions fundamental to whole areas of biology, and in this respect cestodes can be regarded as experimental models for the investigation of basic biological problems and are so regarded in this text. Problems of special interest are the active trans-

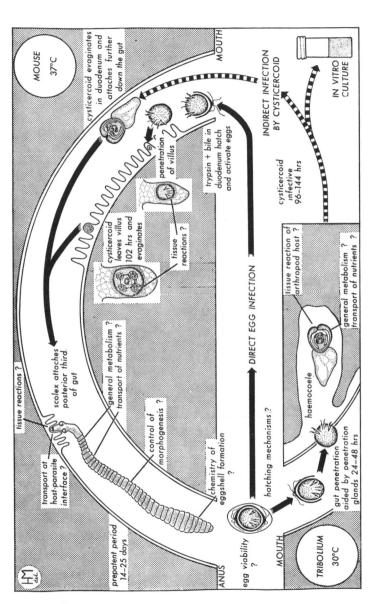

FIG. 1. Life cycle of the rodent cestode, *Hymenolepis nana,* and the physiological problems associated with it. (Original.)

port of materials across the tegument; the factors controlling growth and differentiation of the strobila; the nature and formation of the egg and its protective capsule; the physico-chemical factors stimulating the hatching of the egg in the intermediate host; the role of mechanical and enzymatic factors in penetrating the gut wall; the factors controlling differentiation of the larvae and the immunological relationships of all stages with their hosts. The relationship of some of these problems to the life cycle, with reference to *Hymenolepis nana* is shown in Fig. 1.

A feature of the research carried out on cestode physiology is the small number of species which have been used for experimental purposes, the great majority of work having been carried out on the *Hymenolepis diminuta*, *H. nana*, *Taenia* spp., *Moniezia* spp. and *Echinococcus* spp. amongst the Cyclophyllidea, and various species of the Diphyllobothriidae among the Pseudophyllidea.

The use of these particular species has undoubtedly been due to the relative ease with which they can be maintained in the laboratory or obtained from abattoirs. This does not necessarily mean that the species used represented the *best* experimental material for study of a particular problem; other, but perhaps less readily available, species could serve as better experimental models.

Genetics of the Host-Parasite Relationship

The host-parasite relationship in cestodes is a complex one involving (with rare exceptions) interactions between at least two, and sometimes more, genetical systems, namely those of the parasite, its intermediate and its definitive host. Thus a cestode, if it is to survive, must be suitably adapted to the morphology, physiology, biochemistry, immunology and ecology of its hosts. Unfortunately, speciation in cestodes is still largely defined by workers in terms of gross morphology; but it is clear that all aspects of the biology of a species must be considered if an accurate, integrated picture of its phenotype is to be obtained.

Like trematodes,[422] cestodes have genetical characteristics which make them (theoretically at least!) susceptible to the production of ' strains ' adapted to a new species or ' strains ' of intermediate or definitive host. Thus (*a*) since they are hermaphrodites, an unexpressed recessive mutant gene from one generation will appear in both male and female germ cells at the same time in the P_1 generation; (*b*) self-fertilisation of a proglottid may occur in some cases, or if cross-fertilisation between proglottids of adjacent worms does occur, it is likely—on ecological and behavioural grounds—that mating individuals will have closely related (if not identical) genotypes. Thus, a single mutation could give rise to a homozygous double recessive and an 'instant' mutant could appear.[433] Since the larvae of certain genera (e.g. *Echinococcus*, *Multiceps*) multiply by polyembryony (i.e. asexual multiplication of the original embryo), enormous numbers of new individuals of the new 'mutant' strain could theoretically appear simultaneously, in some cases. Consider for example, a heterozygous worm ($R\ r$) carrying a recessive gene r. Since the reproductive system is hermaphrodite,

$$\text{selfing} = \overset{\male}{Rr} \times \overset{\female}{Rr};$$

therefore F_1 genotypes $= RR$, $2Rr$, rr (eggs).

Suppose, when eggs are ingested by an intermediate host, only those of genotype rr are metabolically or immunologically adapted to the host. Consequently, only rr develops to larva: polyembryony gives a clone of genetically identical individuals. Therefore a new 'strain' is developed.

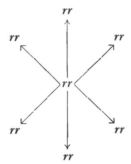

There is increasing evidence in the genus *Echinococcus*, at least,[421] that such strains occur in different hosts; and similar 'strains' of other cestode species may be more widespread than at present believed. Since physiologically and biochemically different strains of both parasite and host can occur, it is important that this fact be given due weight when considering the biology of apparently morphologically identical cestode 'species'.

2: The Adult Cestode: Special Structural Features Relevant to its Physiology

The Tegument

General Remarks

It has already been emphasised (p. 1) that the body-covering of cestodes is a metabolically active surface which plays an extremely important role in their physiology. Although the dynamic nature of this layer is now generally recognised, this was not always the position, for electron mioscopy has virtually revolutionised our knowledge of this region. Moreover, such studies have revealed that in all the groups of parasitic platyhelminths, this layer shows a remarkable degree of uniformity. This observation came as something of a surprise to parasitologists, who had long regarded the ' cuticle ' of cestodes and that of trematodes as different structures. Moreover, studies with labile compounds have shown that trematodes—like cestodes—can take in materials directly through the body wall[422]; morphological similarity between these groups is thus reflected in a similar type of physiological behaviour.

The origins of the platyhelminth ' cuticle ' have long been a matter of dispute[216, 422]; that of cestodes being formerly considered to be made up of inert material secreted from the subcuticular cells.[179, 471] Early ultrastructure studies identified mitochondria in the ' cuticle ' of *Hymenolepis diminuta*, thus indicating that this structure was not inert but cytoplasmic in nature. Since the term ' cuticle ' implied a tough, resistant inert covering, the term ' tegument' was suggested as being more appropriate[337] and this term has been widely adopted. The structure of the helminth ' cuticle' (= tegument) has been reviewed in detail by Lee.[216]

Ultrastructure

(a) *General account.* Most of the work on the ultrastructure of the tegument of adult cestodes has been carried out on the Cyclophyllidea; of these the following species have been examined: *Hymenolepis diminuta;*

H. nana[193, 227, 301, 335, 337, 340, 341]; *Moniezia expa*·*tsa*[172]; *Raillietina cesticillus*[193, 301]; *Anomotaenia constricta*[23]; *Dipylidium caninum*[454]; *Taenia pisiformis; T. hydatigena; Echinococcus granulosus.*[183, 247, 250] Of the other groups, the following have been examined, *Caryophyllaeus* spp.[23]; *Schistocephalus solidus*[456] (Pseudophyllidea); *Proteocephalus pollanicoli*[455] (Proteocephaloidea); *Lacistorhynchus tenuis*[227, 228] (Trypanorhyncha); *Calliobothrium verticillatum*[227] (Tetraphyllidea).

The ultrastructure of the larval stages of the following have also been examined: *Multiceps serialis*[212, 293]; *S. solidus*[233, 456]; *E. granulosus*[247, 251, 428]; *T. pisiformis.*[247]

As with most ultrastructure studies, each year sees improvements in technique, so that the more recent work should provide an increasingly reliable picture of the structures involved.

It is now possible to present a generalised picture of the cestode tegument which is revealed—not as a non-living secreted layer as believed by earlier microscopists—but as a metabolically active, syncytial, protoplasmic layer. This layer is formed by cytoplasmic extensions from tegumental cells lying in the ' sub-cuticular zone ' of classical microscopy (Figs. 2, 3). This zone is separated from the outermost layer by a prominent basement membrane. It is convenient to use the terms applied to trematodes[49, 422]—namely *distal cytoplasm* (= cuticular matrix) for the surface syncytium and '*perinuclear cytoplasm* ' for the cytoplasm in the region of tegumental cells (= subcuticular cells) lying in the subcuticle from which they arise. Continuity between the distal and perinuclear cytoplasm is maintained by narrow cytoplasmic connections (Fig. 2).

Under light microscopy, the free surface of the distal cytoplasm appears as a fringe of fine hair-like processes. At the electron microscope level, these are revealed as a series of spine-like processes which morphologically resemble the brush border of many vertebrate and invertebrate cells and have been referred to as *microvilli*,[23, 216] *tegumental projections*,[250] or *microtriches*.[337] They are referred to here as microtriches (singular, ' microthrix ') and their fine structure is further considered below.

(*b*) *The microtriches.* Microtriches generally cover the scolex and suckers, but may be much reduced or missing altogether from certain areas.[335, 341] The size of the microtriches varies greatly between species. In *H. diminuta* they are 750 mμ in length (on the strobila), but in *Lacistorhynchus* and *Calliobothrium* may reach 2·0 μ.[227] Each microthrix (Fig. 4) consists essentially of a shaft borne on a less dense proximal base. In some cestodes the microtriches appear round in transverse section[227] although in *Echinococcus* they are rhomboid or polyhedral at the base of the shaft.[183]

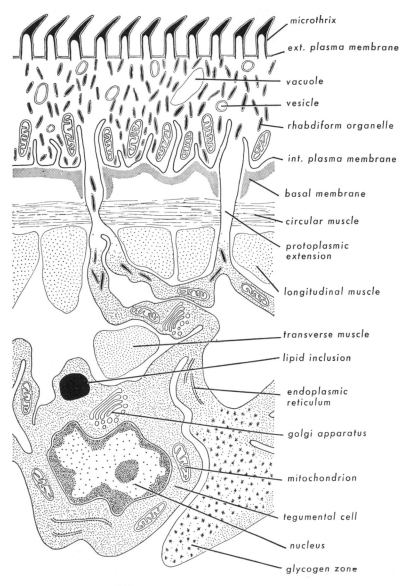

FIG. 2. Ultrastructure of the tegument of *Caryophyllaeus laticeps* (Pseudophyllidea). (After Béguin, 1966.)

Most workers have described microtriches as covered with an outer 'double' membrane continuous with the limiting membrane of the distal cytoplasm.[23, 227, 250]   Studies on *Echinococcus* at higher resolutions suggest that the structure of microtriches appears to be more complicated than was previously thought[183] in that: (*a*) two 'double' (=unit?) membranes, an outer and inner one, cover a microthrix; (*b*) gaps or

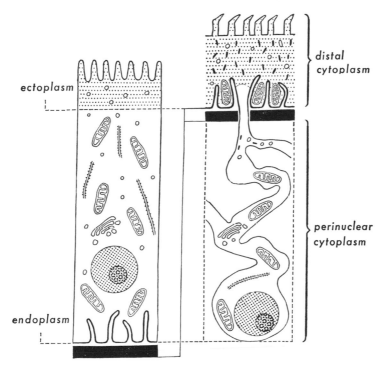

INTESTINAL CELL   CESTODE TEGUMENT

FIG. 3. Structural analogy between the tegumental cells of cestodes (*right*) and the epithelial cells of the vertebrate intestine (*left*). (After Béguin, 1966.)

discontinuities are revealed in the outer plasma membrane in both longitudinal and transverse sections (Frontispiece; Figs. 4, 5); and (*c*) microtubules are revealed to be present in the core of the shaft.

The outer microthrix membrane in *Echinococcus* consists of a membrane, 115–145 Å thick, made up of two electron dense layers, each 40–55 Å thick, and a gap of 40–60 Å between the two.   Tangential sections of this membrane reveal a hexagonal pattern (Fig. 5). These observations have been interpreted[183] as the plasma membrane of a microthrix being modified into a regular 'tubework' with hexagonal spaces between, as is shown diagrammatically in Fig. 5. The shaft, or main body, of a microthrix is limited by a second continuous 'double' (= unit ?) membrane inside the outer membrane structure. The units of each 'double' membrane covering a microthrix show a remarkable globular structure (Fig. 4). This pattern has been associated with membranes concerned with particular enzyme functions (e.g. mito-

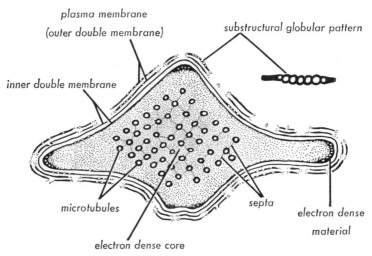

FIG. 4. Diagrammatic interpretation of the ultrastructure of a microthrix of *Echinococcus granulosus* as seen in cross section; the 'double' membranes may prove to be modified unit membranes. (After Jha & Smyth, 1969.)

chrondrial membranes[395]) and may indicate release of enzymes associated with 'membrane digestion' (p. 90) at the host-parasite interface. It has also been shown that the inner core of the shaft contains *microtubules* each with a diameter of about 95–105 Å and a wall about 30–35 Å thick.[183] These microtubules run parallel to the longitudinal axis of a microthrix and appear to be joined together by means of electron-dense septa in a roughly hexagonal manner. These microtubules are probably identical with the parallel 'fibrils' described in *Caryophyllaeus*[23] and *Hymenolepis*[227] Similar types of microtubules have been seen in the microvilli of intestinal epithelium in mice[264] and may prove to be related to the absorptive nature of that structure. It would thus appear that morphologically the tegument of cestodes is beautifully adapted for its function. The spine-like nature of the microtriches would undoubtedly assist in maintaining the position of a worm in the gut, and the surface of the exposed microtriches, with their contained microtubules, pressed into the mucosa, would offer an extensive area for absorption and secretion.

The extent to which the microtriches increase the possible surface for absorption (and/or secretion, p. 13) has been approximately calculated for *Caryophyllaeus* and *Anomotaenia*[23] (Table 1).

If L = length of microthrix (proximal cylindrical region),
d = diameter of microthrix (= $2r$),
B = area of insertion,
n = number of microtriches per μ^2,

Then ratio (R_1) of surface of a microthrix to surface of insertion is:

$$R_1 = \frac{2\pi r L}{\pi r^2} = \frac{2L}{r} = \frac{4L}{d};$$

from which the relation of actual surface area to a corresponding area devoid of villi is:

$$R_2 = \frac{1 - nB + nBR_1}{1} = 1 + nB\,(R_1 - 1).$$

Results are shown in Table 1. Rather surprisingly, it can be seen that microtriches appear to increase the surface area by only 3–6 times,

TABLE 1

Relative increase in surface area of tegument of cestodes, due to microtriches, compared with increase in area of intestine of mouse and Ascaris *due to microvilli ; see pp.* 10–11 *(After Béguin.[23])*

Material	L/d	R_1	$B(\mu^2)$	n	R_2
Caryophyllaeus laticeps	1·3	5·2	0·03	16	3·1
Caryophyllaeus fennica	5·4	21·6	0·01	25	6·1
Anomotaenia constricta	1·8	7·2	0·06	9	4·1
Small intestine of mouse	8·0	32	0·01	80	26
Intestine of *Ascaris*	8·0	320	0·01	40	129

compared with 26 times for microvilli in the mouse intestine and 126 times in the intestine of *Ascaris*.[23] Such a figure does not, however, take into account the modified structure of the plasma membrane as exemplified by the surface mosaic (Fig. 5).

(c) *The Distal and Perinuclear Cytoplasm.* It is evident that in morphology and function, the tegument cells bear a striking resemblance to intestinal mucosa cells (Fig. 3). When the fine structure of

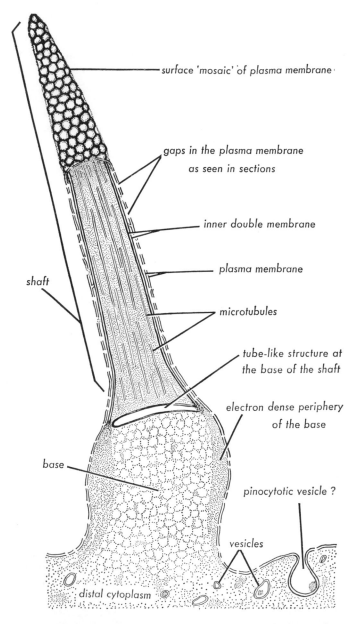

surface 'mosaic' of plasma membrane

gaps in the plasma membrane
as seen in sections

inner double membrane

plasma membrane

shaft

microtubules

tube-like structure at
the base of the shaft

electron dense periphery
of the base

base

pinocytotic vesicle ?

vesicles

distal cytoplasm

FIG. 5. Diagrammatic interpretation of the ultrastructure of a microthrix of *Echinococcus granulosus* as seen in vertical section; see legend, Fig. 4. (After Jha & Smyth, 1969.)

the distal and perinuclear cytoplasm is examined, however, the cells making up these regions can also be seen to resemble cells which are engaged in the synthesis and secretion of protein, such as mammalian pancreatic acinar cells.[227]

Thus, the distal cytoplasm contains numerous organelles containing varying amounts of electron-dense material, each bounded by a 'double' membrane. The terms *vesicles*, *vacuoles* and *rhabdiform organelles* (Fig. 2) have been used for these structures. Mitochondria also occur in the distal and perinuclear cytoplasm, but their numbers appear to vary with species. In *Calliobothrium*,[227] for example, they are rare, but they are numerous in *H. diminuta*. In general, cestode mitochondria have fewer cristae than are typically encountered in aerobic tissue,[230] and this probably reflects the largely anaerobic character of the metabolism (Chapters 4, 5). It has also been suggested that in cestodes, mitochondrial synthesis of nucleoside phosphate esters is largely ' uncoupled ' from aerobic respiration; CO_2 fixation (p. 76) may also take place—at least partially—in the mitochondria.[230]

The Golgi apparatus is situated in the juxtanuclear cytoplasm (Fig. 2), and is surrounded by numerous vesicles which appear in intimate association with the ribosome-rich cisternae of the endoplasmic reticulum. This is a condition associated with a cell actively synthesising protein. Studies with labelled amino acids[229] indicate high levels of protein synthetic activity in the perinuclear cytoplasm and subsequent secretion of the products into the distal cytoplasm. It is not yet known if these products are ultimately released at the surface. Although the structure of this secretion (or secretions) is not known, it may prove to be (an) enzyme(s), for a number of enzymes have been identified in the tegument (Table 2); or again, it may contribute to the amorphous (polysaccharide) coating covering the external plasma membrane; this covering corresponds to the PAS-positive layer of light microscopy. If some of the secretory products proved to be proteolytic enzymes, this would fit in with the view (p. 90) that ' membrane digestion ' occurs at or in the host-parasite interface, although its relation to apparent enzymatic activity of the outer membranes of the microtriches is not clear.

There is some descriptive evidence that pinocytic activity occurs at the integumental surface, and numerous authors have described vacuole-like structures which appear to arise pinocytotically in the external plasma membrane (Fig. 5).[183, 227, 247, 455] Such structures could also be interpreted as indicating release of (enzymatic?) material, so that there is still no unequivocal evidence in support of pinocytosis. Attempts to demonstrate pinocytosis in *Echinococcus* using ferritin, have so far proved unsuccessful.[429]

TABLE 2

Histochemical demonstration of some enzymes in the tegument of cestodes
(+ = present ;   − = absent ;   . = not tested for)

Species	alkaline phosphatase	acid phosphatase	esterase	β-glucuronidase	succinic dehydrogenase	cytochrome oxidase	amylophosphorylase	transglucosidase	References (as numbered in the list)
Anoplocephala magna	+	+	.	.	.	.	.	.	488
Anoplocephala perfoliata	+	+	+	.	.	.	.	.	218, 488
Cysticercus bovis	+	−	.	.	.	.	.	.	489
Cysticercus fasciolaris	+	+	.	.	.	.	.	.	489
Cysticercus tenuicollis	+*	+*	.	.	.	.	.	.	100
Davainea proglottina	+	.	.	.	.	.	.	.	219
Diphyllobothrium mansoni (plerocercoid)	+	+	.	.	.	.	.	.	446
Dipylidium caninum	+	+	−	.	.	.	.	.	363, 470
Echinococcus granulosus	+	−a +b	.	.	.	.	.	.	200[a], 489[b]
Hydatigera (Taenia) taeniaeformis	+	+	+	.	+	.	.	.	217, 343, 363, 469, 470, 488
Hymenolepis citelli	+	−	+	.	+	.	.	.	217, 342, 343
Hymenolepis diminuta (cysticercoid)	.	.	.	.	+	.	.	.	155
Hymenolepis diminuta	+	+	+a −b	−	−	+	−	−	155, 217[a], 343, 363[b], 470
Hymenolepis microstoma	+	+	+	.	+	.	.	.	32, 217, 343
Hymenolepis nana	+	+	−	−	+	+	−	−	363[a], 470
Hymenolepis nana (cysticercoid)	.	.	.	.	+	.	.	.	155
Ligula intestinalis (plerocercoid)	+	+	−	.	.	.	.	.	14
Ligula intestinalis	+	+	−	.	.	.	.	.	14
Moniezia benedeni	+	+	.	.	.	.	.	.	219, 488
Moniezia expansa	+	+	.	.	.	.	.	.	100. 332, 488
Multiceps serialis	+	.	.	.	.	.	.	.	219
Raillietina cesticillus	+	.	.	.	.	.	.	.	219
Taenia pisiformis	+	+	.	.	.	.	.	.	99
Taenia pisiformis (cysticercus)	+*	+*	.	.	.	.	.	.	99
Taenia saginata	+	.	.	.	.	.	.	.	67, 219

* demonstrated by biochemical methods only

The Scolex

General Account

Cestodes live in what might be termed a 'hazardous' environment, in which the peristaltic movement of the gut and the passage of partly digested food make the possession of an efficient form of attachment an essential prerequisite for survival.

The various forms of the cestode scolex or holdfast, are well known, and are described in standard texts.[16, 179, 471] In general, the form of the scolex is beautifully adapted for attachment to the mucosa of a specific host; but some species (e.g. *Ligula intestinalis*), with a poorly developed scolex not specifically adapted to any particular host intestine, have a wide host spectrum.

Although the scolex clearly acts as an organ of attachment, it may in some cestodes, e.g. *Echinococcus*, have a 'placental' function also, i.e. it is able to absorb nutriment from the mucosal wall—a condition known to occur in some trematodes.[422] This view is supported by the fact that in this species the tegument covering each sucker possesses fully developed microtriches.[251]

Form of Adhesive Organs

In general, there are three types of scoleces—the acetabulate, the bothriate and the bothridiate. The *acetabulate* type, which is especially characteristic of the Cyclophyllidea, can be broadly divided into the 'non-penetrative' and the 'penetrative' types although some scoleces fall between these types. In the former, an attached sucker encloses a group of villi, but the scolex does not penetrate deeply into the mucosa. In the 'penetrative' type of scolex, attachment is more intimate and the crypts of Lieberkühn are invaded. In the Taenioidea, this type of scolex typically bears a rostellum—a dome-like or finger-like extension of the scolex—present in such well-known forms as *E. granulosus*, *Dipylidium caninum* and *H. nana*. The rostellum may exist as a permanent extension or as a protrusible organ. In some cases, e.g. *E. granulosus* and *H. nana*, the rostellum carries a muscular rostellar pad (Figs. 6, 12) which presses out the tip of the hooked rostellum, thus making withdrawal difficult. The rostellum in some species is supplied with exocrine glands (see below).

The *bothriate* type of scolex consists typically of a pair of shallow elongate sucking grooves. Each bothrium may take the form of a groove, slit or saucer or, by fusion of the margins, a tube. In some pseudophyllids, e.g. *Ligula* and *Schistocephalus*, the bothria occur as shallow grooves which can have little, if any, attachment function. Both species have markedly progenetic plerocercoids and maturation is accomplished within 36–72 hours (p. 169)—an adaptation undoubtedly related to the weak mode of attachment and the associated difficulty of maintaining a position in the gut.

The *bothridiate* type of scolex is characteristic of the Tetraphyllidea, and typically bears four leaf-like outgrowths or bothridia (phyllidea) whose morphology is closely adapted to that of its host's mucosa (p. 26).[483]

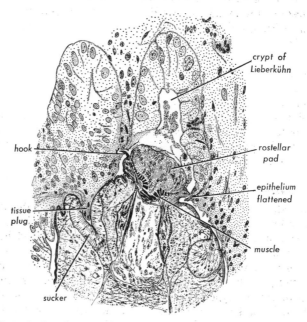

FIG. 6. Attachment of the scolex of *Hymenolepis nana* to the intestine of a mouse. (Original.)

In addition to the adhesive apparatus, many scoleces may be armed with hooks; in the tetrarhynchid cestodes four retractable spiney proboscoides may be protruded. In some instances (e.g. *Spathebothrium*) there is no scolex or any other form of attachment, and in some (e.g. *Parabothrium gadi-pollachi*) the scolex degenerates to form a 'scolex deformatus'. In this species a bulbous swelling at the base of this structure, apparently serves to wedge the anterior end into the caecal wall.[482]

Some tetraphyllids (e.g. *Echeneibothrium maculatum*) possess a large protrusible muscular mass or *myzorhynchus*. Although this again appears to act as an ancillary organ of attachment, it may have a nutritive (i.e. placental) function. Alternatively, or additionally, the fact that it contains a well-developed nerve mass may indicate a sensory function. It would be especially interesting to examine the histochemistry and ultrastructure of this organ.

Glands

Scolex glands. In spite of the obvious importance of the scolex to the physiology of a cestode, surprisingly little is known concerning its cytology and ultrastructure. The fact that gland cells occur in the scolex of many species suggests that this organ is sometimes more than merely an organ of attachment.

In the Pseudophyllidea, glands have been reported in *Diphyllobothrium* spp., *Glandicephalus antarcticus*, *Adinocephalus pacificus* and *Abothrium gadi*.[103, 482] In the Aporidea, the rostellum of *Nematoparataenia southwelli* contains a composite glandular mass which contains three types of cells with different staining reactions.[103] In the Tetraphyllidea, a 'deeply staining mass' has been reported in the scolex of *Monorgyma perfectum*, and in the Lecanicephala a similar 'glandular complex' has been described in *Polypocephalus* spp.[103] In the Cyclophyllidea, glands have been reported in the rostellum of a number of species. In at least one species, *Hymenolepis glandularis*, the glands are extensive and occupy a substantial area of the rostellum. The gland cells are PAS-positive in *T. solium*,[103] *Davainea proglottina*[397] and *Aploparaxis furcigera*.[398]

In *E. granulosus*, gland cells containing drops of secretion occur in the anterior tip of the rostellum. This secretion has proved to be unusually labile and chemically unreactive.[420] Histochemical evidence points to its being a lipoprotein; unlike the secretion of the species mentioned above, it is not PAS-positive. It is also unusual in that it originates in the nucleus of the rostellar gland cell.[432]

If an adult *Echinococcus* is placed in 'immune' canine serum (p. 208), the secretion apparently reacts with antibody and becomes visualised Plate IV.D; Fig. 85.c).[429]

Interproglottidal Glands. Species of the genus *Moniezia* contain extensive *interproglottidal* glands. The glands, which number 6–38, occur in a row along the interproglottidal region. Although the function of these glands is at present unknown, unlike those in the scolex of *Echinococcus*, they are PAS-positive.[392]

Excretory System

The cestode excretory system is based on the platyhelminth protonephridial system with flame cells and collecting vessels; 2–4 longitudinal collecting vessels are common, but up to 20 may occur.[179] In the pseudophyllids, *Ligula* and *Schistocephalus*, there is—in addition to some 16 longitudinal canals—a complex network of vessels situated in the cortical mesenchyme between the subcuticular and mesenchymal systems.   Flame cells of the protonephridial system occur in any part of the body, even in the central nervous system.[384]

Although some of the end products of metabolism are known (pp. 68, 95) and presumably excreted to the outside, the basic physiology of excretion in cestodes has not been closely examined.

Reproductive System

The male system follows the typical platyhelminth pattern with testes, vasa efferentia, vas deferens and cirrus. Protandry—ripening of the male organs before the female—appears to be common among cestodes, although the early stages of maturation have been examined in only a few species.

The female system consists of ovary, oviduct, vagina and uterus. A number of different types of eggs are formed, and the morphology and histochemistry of the genitalia are related to the egg-type produced. For this reason, the morphology of the reproductive system is dealt with in detail later (Chapter 7), when the physiology of egg-formation is considered.

Hermaphroditism is general among cestodes; an exception is the genus *Dioecocestus*, in which the sexes are separate. ' Intersexuality ' occurs in this genus and female organs have been reported in some males.[471] Whether this intersexuality has a genetic and/or an endocrine basis is not known.

Strobilisation of cestodes represents a remarkable phenomenon, for it results essentially in the production of a series of embryos showing increasing degrees of development.   This provides unusual material for experimental embryology, although it has been little utilised as such, except for some studies on the effects of X-radiation.[368]

Muscular System

As in other platyhelminths, the muscular system in cestodes consists of a subcuticular muscle layer and mesenchymal musculature. Morphological descriptions of musculature are given in standard texts[179, 471] and detailed studies of the form and function of several species (e.g. *Bothriocephalus scorpii*, *Clestobothrium crassiceps*,[319] *Echinobothrium brachysoma*, *E. affine*[320] and *Acanthobothrium coronatum*[323] have been made.

The ultrastructure of cestode muscle has been studied in several species.[231] The contractile part of a muscle cell consists of single elongate myofibre, sometimes branched; the myofibre contains thick and thin myofilaments. Microtubules are also present.

The physiology and biochemistry of contraction and relaxation of cestode muscle has scarcely been studied. The motor reactions of the strobila and scolex of *H. nana* have been observed by cinematography and the movements of the scolex, rostellum, suckers and strobila described.[344] It has been shown in *H. nana* that decapitated worms or strobila fragments continue to show waves of contraction for a long time. This suggests that the excitation inducing the waves does not always depend on stimulation from the scolex but appears to be controlled by local stimuli associated with muscle elements.[344]

The attachment of the scolex to the gut raises interesting physiological problems; for the suckers must be in a constant state of contraction and the eversion of the rostellum (when present) must be maintained. Two possible mechanisms for the maintenance of this contraction could be put forward. The first is that adhesive organs are composed of ' catch muscles ' (like those of lamellibranchs), which require little or no energy to maintain them in a state of contraction. Such muscles depend for their functioning on the presence of a special protein component termed ' paramyosin ' especially characterised by having a periodicity of 145 Å.[118a] No attempt appears to have been made to examine cestode muscle for this material, so that it is not known if ' catch muscles ' occur in cestodes. The second possible mechanism involves special nerve cells, termed ' stretch receptors '; these are discussed below (p. 21).

Nervous System

General Account

The nervous system in cestodes has proved exceedingly difficult to study, the difficulty being due chiefly to the lack of a delimiting sheath on the nerve trunks, and to the subsequent problems of demonstrating the nerves by routine staining methods.[385] The use of histochemical methods, based on the demonstration of cholinesterases, however, has revolutionised the study of platyhelminth nervous system. When combined with suitable fixation methods, and appropriately modified, these methods can produce remarkably clear pictures of the nervous system[144, 380] (Plate I). The acetylthiocholine iodide technique[188] and the indoxyl acetate method, as used for trematodes,[422] give the best results; but the lability of the enzymes may vary considerably with species.[380]

Characteristically, the nervous system consists of paired cerebral ganglia united by commissures in the scolex, and lateral longitudinal nerve cords consisting of unmyelinated fibres[252] and also united by commissures, running the length of the strobila. Nerves extend from this system to the muscles, skin and reproductive systems. The interproglottid commissures show up particularly well with the indoxyl acetate technique (Plate I, Fig. B).

The cytology of the nervous system has been little studied. Although various ganglionic cells have been identified in the cerebral ganglia, these appear to be confined mainly to the commissures. In some species, e.g. *Acanthobothrium coronatum* the cerebral 'ganglia' contain no ganglion cells, and this gives some support to an older view that the main nerves and commissures essentially constitute the nervous system. It is much more probable, however, that the scolex, which is the only permanent part of the organism, contains the nerve centre.[321] The synaptic junctions of cestodes do not appear to differ significantly from the characteristic vertebrate and invertebrate type.[252]

Neurosecretory Cells

Neurosecretion is well known in other invertebrates, including the Turbellaria and the Trematoda[422] and has recently been described in *H. diminuta* in sensory bipolar cells located in a cluster in the rostellum.[91a] In the cysticercoid, these cells appear to be inactive and do not stain with paraldehyde-fuchsin, which characteristically (but not specifically) stains neurosecretory material. Granules of fuchsinophilic material appear first in the axons of worms 16–18 days post-infection, but the secretion ceases at 40 days post-infection.[91a] Since the neurosecretory cells first show activity just before strobilisation commences, it can be speculated that these two processes are interrelated. Dense vesicles resembling neurosecretory vesicles have been also described in the nerve processes and in a presumed neuromuscular junction in *E. granulosus*.[252]

Sensory Receptors

Sensory endings which terminate in the tegument have been reported in a number of cestodes, and may be readily demonstrated by histochemical means.[217, 380] Ultrastructure studies have shown that the endings are bulb-like with elongated distal processes extending beyond the tegumental surface (Fig. 7).[252] Morphologically, these resemble those reported from other invertebrates and do not appear to have any unusual features.

Stretch Receptors

As stated earlier (p. 19) in order to maintain the attachment of a
scolex to the mucosa it is probable that the suckers must be maintained

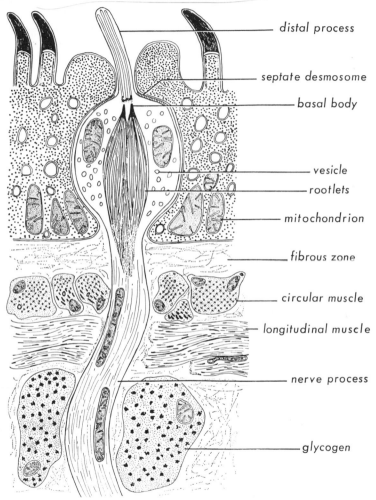

FIG. 7. Schematic diagram of a longitudinal section through a
sensory ending in the tegument of *Echinococcus granulosus*.
(After Morseth, 1967b.)

in a state of more or less continuous contraction. How this is achieved
is not known, but it has been speculated that the action of special

receptors termed 'stretch receptors' may be involved.[321]   These are receptors (best known in crustacea) which have their dendrites deeply embedded in a muscle mass; stretch produces deformation of the dendritic endings with subsequent changes in sensory frequency. The evidence for the existence of stretch receptors in cestodes is, at present, entirely histological and is based on observations of cells, morphologically resembling crustacean stretch receptors in association with the muscles and nerve cords of *Acanthobothrium*.[321]   It will be interesting to see if their presence is confirmed in other species.

Rees[321] speculates that the mechanism of attachment could be as follows.

(a) Tegumental receptors are stimulated on surface contact with the gut, and the stimuli pass to the central nervous system and hence, via motor fibres, to the muscles of the adhesive organs.

(b) The adhesive organs contract and the worm becomes attached.

(c) Contraction of the muscle distorts the dendrites of the stretch receptor, thus initiating an impulse which passes to the nerve cord.

(d) As long as the scolex remains attached to the mucosa, the stimulus persists and the muscle remains contracted. In addition, the action may be modulated by inhibitory fibres from the nerve cord which synapse on either the muscles or the dendrites of the receptors.

An alternative explanation for sustained contraction is that a 'catch muscle' mechanism is involved. This view has been discussed earlier (p. 19).

Transmitter Substances

The identification of possible transmitter substances depends on their biochemical and/or histochemical demonstration, and on the comparative pharmacological effects of extracts of cestodes on other nerve-muscle preparations (such as a leech) and the effects of excitatory or blocking drugs on cestode reactions. Only a very few species have been investigated. The evidence for the existence of acetylcholine—and hence of cholinergic fibres—is as follows.

(a) Cholinesterase has been detected by chemical or histochemical methods in the following species: *D. latum*,[291] *T. saginata*, *Hydatigera taeniaeformis* (*T. crassicolis*), *Hymenolepis* spp.,[15a, 133, 217, 363] *E. granulosus*,[373, 374] *Dipylidium caninum*[15a, 363, 380] (Plate I, Fig. B).

(b) Acetylcholine-like substances, which stimulate leech muscle or inhibit frog's heart, are present in cestode extracts.[15a]

(c) Synthetic acetylcholine accelerates, and then reduces, activity in *H. nana*.[345]

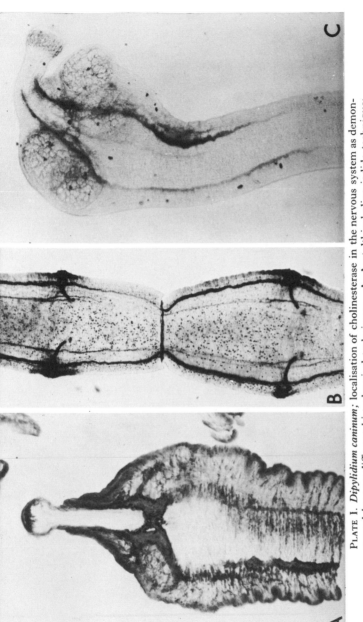

PLATE 1. *Dipylidium caninum*; localisation of cholinesterase in the nervous system as demonstrated by two different histochemical techniques. A. Acetylthiocholine iodide technique; scolex with rostellum extended; frozen section. B. Indoxyl acetate technique; ripe proglottids showing concentration of cholinesterase in genital pore and ducts. C. Indoxyl acetate technique; scolex with rostellum extended; note ganglia in each sucker. (After Shield, 1969.)

(*d*) Eserine, which inhibits cholinesterase, stimulates activity in *D. caninum* on standing.[15a]

There is also some rather inconclusive evidence that adrenergic fibres may be present. This possibility has been investigated only in *H. nana*, and is based on:

(*a*) Adrenaline stimulates the contraction of the strobilus of *H. nana*; this contraction is followed by relaxation and

(*b*) Influence of adrenaline is increased by ephedrine.[345]

Catechol amines have not yet been identified chemically in cestodes; although this could be attempted chemically by paper chromatography, or histochemically by fluorescent microscopy. It is clear that this system requires further extensive investigation.

Electrophysiology

The electrophysiology of cestode nerves has not been the subject of any investigations, and this, again, is an area of cestode physiology which calls for further study.

3: The Adult Cestode in its Environment

General Considerations

As was pointed out earlier, cestodes differ markedly from trematodes and nematodes in that the adults, with a few exceptions, occupy virtually a single type of environmental niche—the alimentary canal. Even the exceptions occur in sites related to the alimentary canal. Examples of some aberrant genera are; *Stilesia*, *Thysanosoma* (bile ducts of sheep), *Porogynia* (bile ducts of guinea-fowl), *Atriotaenia* (pancreatic ducts of *Nasua*), *Progamotaenia*, *Hepatotaenia* (bile ducts, gall bladder and liver of marsupials). Most of these could be classified as exotic species unsuitable for laboratory use. However, *Hymenolepis microstoma*, which occurs in the bile ducts of rodents and which can be successfully reared in the rat and the hamster,[221] is a useful laboratory model.

The anatomy and physiology of the alimentary canal is thus of particular importance to the study of cestode physiology. A number of useful reviews on this topic are available.[91, 379, 403, 404, 486, 487] The bulk of data relates to the alimentary tract of domestic animals and man; few studies on the alimentary canal of other groups of vertebrates or invertebrates appear to have been made. The vertebrate alimentary canal, considered specifically as an environment for parasitic helminths, has received some attention.[296, 334, 417]

The Alimentary Canal as a Biotope

General Morphology

It is not intended to give here a detailed description of the vertebrate alimentary canal, accounts of which are given in the reviews referred to above. Some parameters of the intestinal environment which are likely to be important for the establishment of a cestode are shown in Fig. 8. They are discussed further in Chapter 10. It is important, however, to appreciate that the physiology of a particular species of cestode is

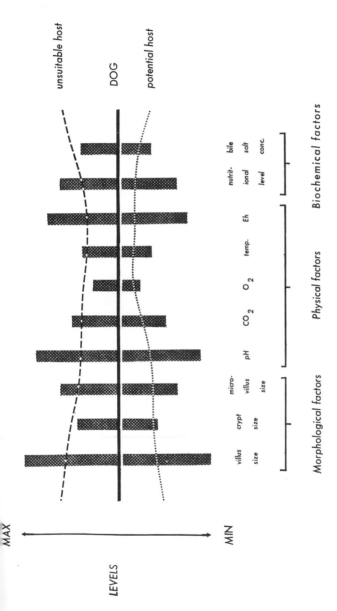

Developmental requirements for Echinococcus granulosus

Fig. 8. Some parameters of the intestinal environment which play a part in the determination of the host specificity of a cestode; based on *Echinococcus granulosus*. The levels of the various factors are only notional, as the limits of tolerance have not been precisely defined. A host intestine with levels outside those shown cannot provide a suitable environment for establishment and growth. (After Smyth & Smyth, 1968.)

likely to be related, not only to the physico-chemical conditions within the gut, but also the the actual topography of the gut surface and the nature of its related glands.   This question, which may be termed micro-ecology, has not, with a few exceptions,[319, 320, 434, 482-4] received much attention in cestodes.   It does not appear to be generally appreciated that, even in closely related hosts, the microstructure of the alimentary canal may show variation in such characteristics as the size of the villi, and the width and depth of crypts—characters which may

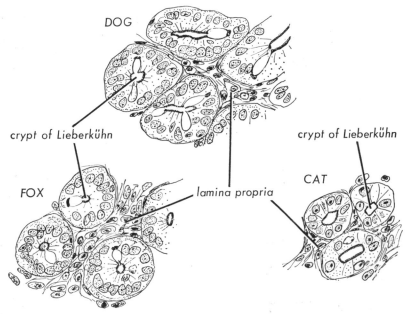

FIG. 9. Comparative size of the crypts of Lieberkühn of three carnivores, as seen in transverse section. (After Smyth & Smyth, 1968.)

be important for the attachment and survival of a cestode.   These characters thus, could clearly play a part in determining host specificity, and evidence is accumulating that the morphology of the scolex in a particular species is very closely adapted to the gut of its host.   This is perhaps best seen in fish hosts such as *Raja montagui, R. clavata* and *R. naevus* whose intestines show considerable morphological variation. Species of the tetraphyllid genus *Echeneibothrium,* which parasitise these hosts, possess scoleces adapted to the depths of the villi, crypts or reticulations of the mucosa in each case.[483]

    Again, the crypt-size of the dog, fox and cat differ substantially (Fig. 9), a fact which may be related to the inability of *Echinococcus granulosus* to grow in the cat or dog, whereas *E. multilocularis* (which is a smaller ' species ') can grow in both these hosts. As was pointed out earlier, other factors, such as the physico-chemical characteristics of the gut, and its immunological reactions, must also, of course, be taken into account (p. 25). The gut-emptying time may also be important.[211]

The general histology of the intestine is too well known to require detailed description here, but attention may be drawn to certain points of particular importance for the study of cestode physiology. A major one of these relates to the mucous lining of the gut. Whereas it has always been recognised that mucosal cells are lost and replaced, the rapidity with which this process takes place was not realised until development of radioactive tracers enabled the dividing cells to be labelled. In all mammals studied, the ' turnover time ' (i.e. the time taken for replacement of the number of cells equal to that in the total population) was found to be less than three days. The turnover time in the duodenum of the rat is 1·6 days, the cat 2·3 days and man 2–6 days.[404] New cells are formed in a crypt and move up along the surface of a villus to the tip as the cells at the tip are cast off. Thus, the contents of the duodenum are continually being supplemented by shed mucosal cells, and the autolysis of these undoubtedly releases a significant amount of nutritional material which would be available to a cestode. Such material undoubtedly plays a part in maintaining the relative constancy of the amino acid ratios in the gut lumen (p. 28). This turnover of mucosal cells may also account for the fact that the immunological responses against adult cestodes are, in general, slight (Chapter 13). Nevertheless, antibodies to helminths have been detected in the mucus of infected hosts (p. 209).

In man, the villi of the small intestine are long finger-like processes, 0·5–1·5 mm in length, which project into the lumen. Studies with special optical instruments passed down the duodenum have revealed that the villi are in constant movement, apparently contracting and relaxing about six times a minute.

Each villus contains an arteriole and a venule with their communicating capillary plexus, and also a lymphatic vessel. The existence of an active blood supply may have physiological significance for a cestode scolex embedded deep in the mucosal wall, especially with regard to the availability of oxygen. Mucus secreted by the goblet cells makes the intestinal surface viscid, a condition which must greatly assist the close adhesion of the tapeworm strobila. This adhesion to the intestinal mucosa is probably essential to the normal nutritional efficiency of cestodes, but the degree of dependence may vary widely with species. At least in *Echinococcus*, as demonstrated by *in vitro* experiments

(p. 182), contact of the scolex with a solid proteinaceous substrate appears to be essential for strobilisation (p. 183).

In vitro experiments, particularly with the pseudophyllidean cestodes *Schistocephalus solidus* and *Ligula intestinalis*, have also demonstrated that, in these species at least, compression of the strobila against a soft surface such as the mucosa is essential for impregnation and fertilisation (p. 169). *E. granulosus* (p. 184) also appears to have some special requirement, as yet unknown, regarding impregnation.

Intestinal Physiology

General comments. As a result of the application of recently developed techniques to intestinal physiology, knowledge of the general digestive processes can be said to have undergone a revolution. Until recently, it was believed that in the gut lumen polysaccharides were broken down to monosaccharides, proteins to amino acids, and fats to glycerol and fatty acids. It was also considered that only the relatively small molecules, produced as a result of these processes, were absorbed by the gut, and that the quantity and proportions of these available at any one time were related to the feeding habits of the host.

Many of these concepts have been challenged, and the evidence[403, 404, 486] now suggests:

(i) that disaccharides can be absorbed by the intestinal mucosa without first being hydrolysed to monosaccharides and that, following absorption, hydrolysis can subsequently take place in the epithelial cells;

(ii) that products of protein digestion larger than amino acids—and possibly whole proteins—can be absorbed;

(iii) that the molar *ratios* of the pool of amino acids in the intestine remain relatively constant, independent of the quantity of the protein ingested in the host diet;[266, 267]

(iv) that the mechanism of transport of amino acids and monosaccharides is not clear, but that it may be carried out by means of ' carriers ' whose nature is not understood.

In relation to (iii) above it must be emphasised that it is the molar *ratios*, not the absolute quantities, of amino acids that remain constant. This effect appears to result from two sources: (*a*) the swamping of ingested proteins by large quantities of protein from digestive secretions, with some contribution from autolysing mucosal cells and (*b*) ' leakage ' of amino acids from the intact epithelium of the mucosal lining.

The full implication of these findings in relation to the physiology of cestodes is not yet apparent, but they clearly have particular relevance to metabolic and *in vitro* studies, and are considered in detail in later chapters.

Absorption mechanisms; *membrane transport*.   The mechanisms, whereby cells, tissues and organs—especially the intestine—absorb substances from their environment, have been a matter of controversy for over seventy years, and it is only within the last few years that the nature of these mechanisms has become somewhat clarified.   The main point at issue has been whether absorption is merely a matter of simple diffusion, or whether some active process, utilising 'secretory' absorptive work, was involved.

The mechanisms of absorption, at present recognised are:

   (i) passive diffusion,
   (ii) active transport,
   (iii) facilitated diffusion (= mediated transport),
   (iv) pinocytosis.

Although it is beyond the scope of this book to deal with these mechanisms in detail, since they probably operate both at the boundary of the cestode environment (i.e. the gut wall) and at the surface of the cestode itself, they have special significance in the studies of cestode physiology.   For this reason they are summarised in outline below.

(i) *Passive diffusion* is the movement of substances across membranes by mechanisms which apparently follow the simple laws of diffusion. In the intestine, passive diffusion appears to be the mechanism of absorption of relatively few materials, among which are water-soluble vitamins, some nucleic acid derivatives, and many lipid-soluble substances.   The rate of movement of a given substance is proportional to the concentration-difference across the membrane, and this relationship can be utilised to test whether this phenomenon is taking place.   The process may be quantitatively described by the Fick equation, which deals with the mass of solute ds diffusing in time dt

$$ds/dt = P \times A(C^{\mathrm{E}} - C^{\mathrm{I}})$$

where P = permeability constant; A = area; C^{E} = external concentration; C^{I} = internal concentration.

The application of Fick's equation to the intestinal epithelium is complicated by the structure of the mucosa.   The surface area is not easily calculated because of the presence of microvilli and the thickness of the epithelial cell, and its basement membrane introduces further difficulties.   Nevertheless, experiments with tied intestinal loops readily demonstrate that Fick's equation holds good for substances such as sorbose (Fig. 10).

(ii) *Active transport*. As the rate of diffusion of most water- and fat-soluble materials is slow, it is not surprising to find that the intestinal mucosa has developed mechanisms which result in the rapid transport of the food materials required for metabolic and synthetic purposes. Salts (e.g. NaCl), glucose, amino acids and fats are all absorbed by such mechanisms. The term 'active transport' has been developed to describe such a mechanism and in recent years has been used to designate ' any process that appears to be inconsistent with the laws of diffusion '.[486] More recently there has been some attempt to restrict the term to ' those

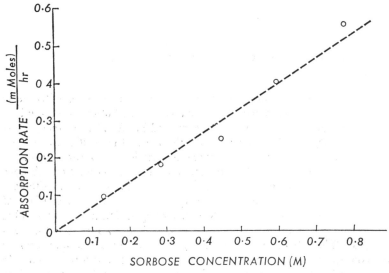

FIG. 10. Effect of concentration on the absorption rate of sorbose by the rat intestine. (After Wilson, 1962.)

processes in which a substance moves across a membrane *against an electrochemical gradient* and consequently requires energy supplied by cellular mechanism '.[486] The process is further characterised by two features: (*a*) it shows stereospecificity, which involves competitive inhibitions by chemically similar compounds; (*b*) it is inhibited by poisons of energy metabolism.

Excellent evidence is now available on the active transport of L-amino acids and sugars and some ions in the intestine, some of these data are listed in Table 3. It is interesting to note that *in vitro* the absorption of glucose by the intestine is dependent on aerobic metabolic pathways and ceases completely under anaerobic conditions (Fig. 11).

As active transport is of importance for the uptake of carbohydrates and amino acids by the cestode cuticle (Chapters 5, 6); the theoretical background to this mechanism is discussed in detail later (p. 102).

(iii) *Facilitated diffusion.* This is a term coined[486] to denote a transport mechanism in which the rate of the attainment of diffusion equilibrium is accelerated without any direct expenditure of energy. It differs from active transport in being unable to operate against an electrochemical gradient. The absorption of D-xylose by the intestine comes under this heading.

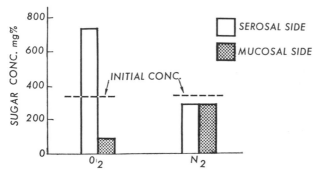

FIG. 11. Active transport of glucose by hamster intestine *in vitro* and its inhibition under anaerobic conditions; everted sacs of intestine incubated with initially the same concentration of glucose on both sides of the gut wall, for 1 hour at 37°C. (After Wilson, 1962.)

(iv) *Pinocytosis.* The ingestion of large particles of food by phagocytosis in *Amoeba* involves the formation in the cell membrane of small channels which separate into small vacuoles termed *pinosomes.* The same phenomenon was later observed in cells in tissue culture and termed *pinocytosis*; and since then it has been described in many tissues. Pinocytosis can be followed by the use of proteins, labelled with fluorescent dyes; these, when taken in by the cell, can be identified by fluorescent microscopy in minute vacuoles in the cytoplasm. Material labelled with radioactive tracers can similarly be used and pinocytosis detected by autoradiography. Pinocytosis has been repeatedly demonstrated in intestinal epithelial cells, and there is no doubt that it plays an important role in absorption of materials. Whether cestodes utilise pinocytosis is not known (p. 13); but, if they do, a cestode could clearly compete with the mucosal cells for food particles of a certain size.

TABLE 3

Active transport of substances by the intestine and location of maximum absorption
(Data from Wilson[486])

Substance	Small intestine			Colon
	Upper*	Mid	Lower	
Absorption				
Sugars (glucose, galactose, etc.)	++	+++	++	o
Neutral amino acids	++	+++	++	o
Basic amino acids	++	++	++	?
Betaine, dimethylglycine, sarcosine	++	++	++	?
Gamma globulin (new born animals)	+	++	+++	?
Pyrimidines (thymine and uracil)	+	+	?	?
Triglycerides	++	++	+	?
Fatty acid absorption and conversion to triglyceride	+++	++	+	o
Bile salts	o	+	+++	.
Vitamin B_{12}	o	+	+++	o
Na^+	+++	++	+++	+++
H^+ (and/or HCO_3^- secretion)	o	+	++	++
Ca^{++}	+++	++	+	?
Fe^{++}	+++	++	+	?
Cl^-	+++	++	+	o
SO_4^-	++	+	o	?
Secretion				
K^+	o	o	+	++
H^+ (and/or HCO^- absorption)	++	+	o	o
Sr^{++}	o	o	+	?
Cl^- (under special conditions)	+	?	?	?
I^-	o	+	o	o

* Upper small intestine refers primarily to jejunum, although the duodenum is similar in most cases studied (with the notable exception that the duodenum secretes HCO_3^- and shows little net absorption or secretion of NaCl).

Physico-chemical Characteristics

(i) *p*H. The *p*H of the alimentary canal has been reviewed by a number of authors[91, 296, 417, 486] and data relative to man and the more common laboratory hosts are available. Results from different workers show some divergence, and the question needs re-examination in some species. It was formerly considered that the *p*H of the duodenum was alkaline, but more recent critical work indicates that it is generally just on the acid side—about 6·7–6·8 (Table 4), but figures as low as 5·1 (in guinea-pig) and as high as 7·8 have been reported. It must be recalled, however, that some cestodes are deeply embedded in the crypts of Lieberkühn, and the pH of this site is not precisely known.   On theoretical grounds, its pH is more likely to approach that of a tissue site than that of the intestinal lumen and is probably close to that of blood (7·4).

TABLE 4

pH and HCO_3^- concentration in intestinal secretions in the dog.   Secretions from Thiry-Vella loops of unanaesthetised dogs, unexposed to air during collection (Data from Wilson[486])

Location	pH	' Total CO_2 ' $(HCO_3^- + CO_2)$ (mm.)
Jejunum	6·8	19
Ileum	7·6	83
Colon	8·0	90

(ii) *Oxidation-reduction potential.*   This characteristic, which may have considerable significance for cestode metabolism (especially in relation to electron transport), has been little studied.   It must be emphasised that the E_h can be influenced by diet or microfloral content —factors which are frequently interrelated.   In the rat, perhaps the best-studied laboratory host, the stomach contents have an E_h value of $+150$ mV, that of the upper and lower small intestine about -100 mV.[166]

(iii) *Oxygen tension.*   The oxygen tension of the vertebrate intestine has long been a matter of interest to parasitologists on account of its significance to the aerobic or anaerobic metabolism of intestinal parasites.   A high O_2 tension in the environment does not necessarily mean that a parasite which lives in such an environment will have an aerobic metabolism.   The trematode *Schistosoma mansoni*, for example, although it lives in the portal blood vessels (an aerobic site) has essentially an anaerobic metabolism.[422]   Respiration in cestodes is discussed later (p. 51).

TABLE 5

The percentage composition of the gases in the small intestine of various vertebrates (Data modified from Read[296])

Animal	CO_2	O_2	CH_4	H_2	N_2
Rabbit	13·56–75	0–0·19	2–2·83	7·72–18	6–75·71
Dog	15·92	0·29	—	26·48	57·28
Goose	2·04–87·83	0–3·62	0–13·51	0·72–20·06	67·92–85·28
Pig	2·16–79·89	0·08–8·2	0–28·29	0–39·56	2·02–92
Horse	15–43	0·57–0·76	0	20–24	37–60
Cattle, sheep and goats	62–92	0	0·04–6·6	0–37	1

Although some oxygen from swallowed air is undoubtedly present in the oesophagus and stomach, the evidence suggests that the oxygen tension drops sharply within the intestine. Some data for the common hosts is given in Tables 5 and 6. The measurement of the oxygen tension is technically not easy, and some early estimations may be open to question.

A figure for the gut of a duck[84] obtained by means of an oxygen electrode implanted in the intestine for some days before recording, probably represents one of the most accurate readings at present available. Figures for one experiment are given in Table 6. The low figures at position zero are thought to result from a reduction in the blood supply to the villi caused by the pressure of the electrode at its deepest position.

TABLE 6

Values of pO_2 in mm Hg found in the lumen of the small intestine of a domestic duck.   Each measurement was repeated three times
(Data from Crompton, Shrimpton & Silver[84])

Time after operation (hr.)	Position of the electrode tip from the intestinal wall. (mm.)				
	0	1	2	3	4
24	<0·5	18·4	5·0	<0·5	<0·5
72	<0·5	17·4	10·0	0	0
168	5·5	<0·5	<0·5	<0·5	<0·5

It is clear from Table 6 and from other experiments, that the oxygen tension approaches zero in the lumen of the gut, but is substantially higher in the region of the mucosa; the highest tension reported in the duck was 25 mm Hg ($= 3·3\% O_2$). This is higher than the figure given (5 mm Hg) as the order of the threshhold for the satisfactory functioning of the enzyme, cytochrome oxidase,[84] (see p. 82). Somewhat comparable results have been found in the rat and sheep, where the layer of liquid immediately in contact with the mucosa has been shown to have tensions of 8–30 mm Hg in the rat, and 4–13 mm Hg in the sheep.[333]

Many cestodes, however, penetrate deep within the crypts of Lieberkühn (Figs. 12, 73), or even break into the lamina propria with the result that they are brought into close contact with blood capillaries, and hence may have access to higher tensions of oxygen than that available in the intestine. It is known that oxygen is essential for evagination of the scolex of *Echinococcus granulosus* and its subsequent development *in vitro*.[423, 430] Since this species has a penetrative type of scolex, this is further indirect evidence that oxygen must be available in the lumen of the crypts. The oxygen tension of dog blood for 95% or more saturation to occur is 75 mm Hg ($= 10\%$ oxygen), and it is likely that the oxygen tension in the crypts approaches this level. On the other hand, *H. nana* can be cultured to maturity in an anaerobic environment.[166, 393] The problem of the amount of oxygen actually available to a cestode may be further complicated by the fact that, since mucosal cells have a very high oxygen requirement,[486] there may be competition between the mucosal epithelial cells and cestode tissue.

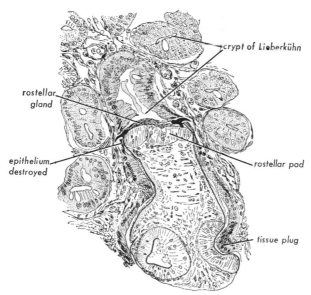

FIG. 12. Scolex of adult *Echinococcus granulosus* in its characteristic position in the duodenum of a dog. The rostellum is extended into a crypt of Lieberkühn with the hooks lightly penetrating the epithelium which has become flattened. See also Fig. 73. (Original.)

(iv) *Presence of other gases.* In addition to oxygen, nitrogen, carbon dioxide and—rather surprisingly—hydrogen, are found in the alimentary canal. The occurrence of hydrogen is unusual and is confined, in any quantity, to the dog (Table 5). The level of CO_2 is important, as there is now firm evidence indicating that CO_2-fixation occurs, and that this gas is a valuable source of carbon atoms to cestodes—at least in some species. The evidence for this is discussed in Chapter 5. The partial pressure of CO_2, i.e. the pCO_2, under standard conditions (760 mm Hg) can be calculated from the equation

$$pCO_2 = \frac{P(CO_2\%)}{760 \times 100} \text{ atmospheres}$$

where $(CO_2\%) = \%CO_2$ at atmospheric pressure P. In dog and man, the pCO_2 probably lies between 5 and 10%,[166] although higher levels have been reported (Table 5).

Bile

General Account. Bile is of particular importance to intestinal parasites, for in many cases it is involved in the ' trigger mechanisms ' concerned in the hatching of helminth eggs, excystation of protozoan cysts, evagination of cestode scoleces, and excystation of trematode metacercaria.[426] In relation to cestodes, its role in egg hatching and scolex evagination is dealt with later (pp. 124 and 146). It has only recently been recognised that the composition of bile varies greatly between species (Tables 7 and 8) and that this difference may play some part in determining host specificity.[416, 426]

TABLE 7
Some quantitative data on the major constituents of bile; analyses in mg/100 ml
(Data from Smyth & Haslewood[426])

	Total lipids	Bilirubin	Cholesterol	Fatty Acids	Total Bile Acid
Ox	100–160	—	37	370	7,200
Dog	—	92–170	80–100	1,600–5,000	7,900–1,500
Guinea pig	140	—	—	—	780
Rabbit	—	87–131	10–120	—	1,100–2,600
Rat*	—	8–3	12·7	—	—
Pig	—	32–62	130–150	820–2,000	8,500–12,000
Man	—	140	430	2,400	11,500

* No gall bladder.

Bile is secreted continuously by the cells of the liver and stored in the gall bladder. In a few mammals, e.g. the rat, a gall bladder is lacking. Although small amounts of bile may enter the alimentary canal regularly, the ingestion of food normally stimulates the emptying of the gall bladder, and bile enters the intestine in quantity during that time. It is important to note that, during the period of storage in the gall bladder, certain substances, such as water and inorganic salts, may be absorbed so that the composition of ' gall bladder bile ' and ' hepatic fistula bile ' may differ substantially.

Chemical composition. Although bile contains pigments, cholesterol, fatty acids, some sugars and bile salts, it is these last that are of particular importance to the physiology of cestodes.

Bile salts are substances, derived from sterols, which make up a substantial part of the solid matter in bile and which play an important part in the intestinal digestive processes probably by virtue of their

TABLE 8

Qualitative data on the composition of bile acids in man and common laboratory and domestic animals

(Data from Smyth & Haslewood[426])

Species	Rate of secretion ml/kg body wt./24 hr.	Bile acids	Nature of conjugation
Man	2·6–15·0	Cholic, chenodeoxycholic, deoxycholic, lithocholic, ursodeoxycholic	Taurine, glycine
Ox	15·4	Cholic, deoxycholic, chenodeoxycholic, lithocholic, 3α-hydroxy-12-oxocholanic, 3α, 12α-dihydroxy-7-oxocholanic, 7α, 12α-dihydroxy-3-oxocholanic, 3α-hydroxyl-7, 12α-dioxocholanic, stereocholic, sapocholic	Taurine, glycine
Sheep	12·1	Cholic, deoxycholic, chenodeoxycholic	Taurine, glycine
Guinea-pig	228	Chenodeoxycholic ; 3α-hydroxy-7-oxocholanic, cholic, ursodeoxycholic	Taurine, glycine
Rabbit	118	Deoxycholic, lagodeoxycholic, cholic, lithocholic	Glycine
Fox	?	Cholic, deoxycholic	Taurine
Dog	5–52	cholic, deoxycholic, chenodeoxycholic	Taurine
Cat	14·0	Cholic	Taurine
Rat	28·6–47·1	Cholic, chenodeoxycholic, ursodeoxycholic, α- and β-muricholic	Taurine, glycine
Mouse	?	Cholic, α- and β-muricholic, chenodeoxycholic	?
Pig	25·2	Cholic, hyocholic, chenodeoxycholic, hyodeoxycholic, 3α, 6 β-dihydroxycholanic, 3β, 6α-dihydroxycholanic, 3α-hydroxy-6-oxocholanic (or allocholanic), lithocholic	Taurine glycine

surface tension lowering properties. The structure and properties of these salts have been reviewed in detail by Haslewood.[146] Bile salts essentially have molecules of the ' detergent ' type with a hydrocarbon, fat-dissolving part and a polar, water-attracting part. The fat-dissolving part consists of the bulk of the steroid nucleus. The hydroxyl groups are so distributed that hydration can readily take place; the remainder of the molecule will dissolve in the fatty phase. Emulsification of fat/water complexes can thus easily occur.

Types of salts. There are three types of bile salts (*a*) C_{27} (or C_{28}) alcohols, (*b*) C_{27} (or C_{28}) acids, and (*c*) C_{24} acids. The alcohols have been isolated only from amphibia and fishes (especially elasmobranchs). The C_{27} (or C_{28}) bile acids are little known, and occur mainly in reptiles. The C_{24} bile acids are better known, and are mostly derived from cholanic acid, $C_{24}H_{40}O_2$. The best known salts are those of cholic acid, hyocholic acid, chenodeoxycholic acid, deoxycholic and litho-cholic acid (Table 8).

Conjugation of bile salts. Bile alcohols and acids normally occur in conjugated forms. Alcohols are conjugated with sulphate giving substances of the type $R: CH.O\text{-}SO_3$. Bile salts conjugate with the amino acids taurine ($NH_2CH_2CH_2SO_3H$) and glycine (NH_2CH_2COOH). In mammals there is a tendency for the salts of herbivorous animals to be conjugated with glycine, and those of carnivorous animals to be conjugated with taurine. This is only a broad generalisation, however, as information on this point is incomplete. Cat and dog bile are almost exclusively conjugated with taurine, whereas rabbit bile acids are almost exclusively conjugated with glycine.

As will be shown later (p. 147), the cestode tegument of certain species is especially sensitive to some bile salts—especially deoxycholic acid—which lyse it at certain concentrations.

Osmotic Relationships

The osmotic relationships of cestodes have been reviewed.[316] Although a number of observations have been made on individual species, insufficient accurate information has been produced to enable a reliable generalisation to be made. Some of the earlier work in this field may be open to criticism on the grounds that it was carried out by methods no longer acceptable. Many worms appear to behave like osmometers, and when placed in an environment with a different osmotic pressure can only adjust their internal osmotic pressure by varying their body volume. *Moniezia*,[316] *Hymenolepis*,[57] *Schistocephalus*,[405] and *Calliobothrium*[308] change their wet weight almost arithmetically in response to a change in external osmotic pressure (Fig. 13).

The question of the osmotic relationship between a cestode and its environment is complicated by the discoveries of methods of passage of substances through membranes by means other than diffusion (p. 29). These principles apply not only to the intestinal mucosa but also to the cestode tissue (see p. 90). Hence, the actual osmotic pressure of a solution as measured by physico-chemical means may not be as significant to a worm as the actual content of materials to which the tegument of the worm is 'permeable'—using the word in its widest sense as indicated above. The reason for this is that substances in the medium which (theoretically) contribute to the total osmotic pressure of the medium, do not actually exert osmotic pressure across the tegument of the worm which separates the worm from its environment.

Thus, differences in 'permeability' of solute can create curious anomalous situations. In the case of the avian cestode, *Tetrabothrius erostris*, both sucrose at 0·192 M (Δ = −0·36°C) and NaCl at 0·140 M

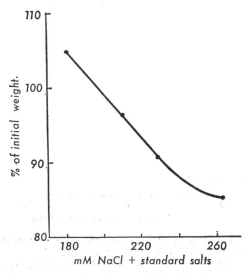

Fig. 13. Change in wet weight of *Calliobothrium verticillatum* after 150 minute incubation in salt solutions in which NaCl was varied. KCl, $MgCl_2$, and $CaCl_2$ were present at standard concentrations in all media. Each curve represents data from 4 to 7 worms. (After Read, Douglas & Simmons, 1959.)

(Δ = − 0·56°C) appear to be isosmotic; this result can be interpreted as showing that this species is less permeable to sucrose than to Na^+ and Cl^- ions.

It is interesting to note that, in the case of cestodes of elasmobranchs, urea—which is well known to contribute substantially to the osmotic pressure of blood in many species of elasmobranchs—occurs in quantity in some cestodes of these fishes. Thus, the tetraphyllidean *Calliobothrium verticillatum* contains urea concentrations of 1·03 ± 0·46% of the wet weight, the equivalent of 3·7% dry weight.[308] When worms were incubated in solutions lacking urea, the urea in the worm tissues rapidly disappeared, but this did not occur if urea was present in the external medium. Similar results were obtained with the tetra-phyllideans *Phyllobothrium foliatum* and *Inermiphyllidium pulvinatum.* Later studies with ^{14}C-labelled urea on the kinetics of urea entry in *C. verticillatum* showed that equilibrium between urea in worm tissues and in the external medium was reached in 60–90 minutes (Fig. 14).

It is surprising to find that *Lacistorhynchus tenuis*, from the same host as *C. verticillatum*, does not behave osmotically in a similar manner. The amount of free urea in this species is low, and later work[391] showed that urea was metabolised by this cestode.

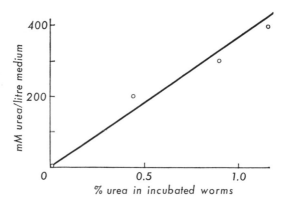

FIG. 14. The urea content of *Calliobothrium verticillatum* as a function of the urea content of the medium. The worms were incubated for 180 minutes in salt solution containing standard concentrations of KCl, $MgCl_2$, and $CaCl_2$ and 190mM of NaCl per litre. Urea was added at the indicated concentrations. Each point represents data from 8 to 12 worms. (After Read, Douglas & Simmonds, 1959.)

The mechanism of the elimination of water or salt is unknown; presumably the flame cells of the excretory system are involved. The mechanism of this system as an osmoregulator does not appear to have been studied. It is interesting to note that the excretory system is the first organ system to become prominent during the early stages of differentiation of the protoscoleces of *Echinococcus* to a strobilate worm in the dog gut. The appearance of this system, may, however, be related to the need to eliminate waste materials with special rapidity during this early period of differentiation. Experiments to demonstrate that the excretory canals are involved in the transportation of absorbed substances from one part of a worm to another, have, so far, been unsuccessful.

4: The Adult: General Metabolism and Chemical Composition; Respiration

General Background

Basic Problems

In biochemical studies on cestodes, one of the most challenging problems is to relate results from studies carried out *in vitro* (often on homogenates), to the processes which actually occur *in vivo*. Thus, the physico-chemical conditions of the system used, especially the pO_2, pCO_2, E_h and pH, are likely to have a profound influence on the chemical reactions *in vitro*; yet these are very imperfectly known for most *in vivo* parasite systems (Chapter 3). Furthermore, *in vitro* test substances may come in contact with metabolically active centres in homogenates, whereas in whole worms permeability factors may prevent effective interaction of these materials. Finally, the spatial distribution of enzymes or substrates in the whole organism may be such that certain enzymes or substrates, which may occur in independent sites (e.g. in the nucleus and in the mitochondria), may never come in contact with one another in the living cell. Under the artificial conditions created within tissue homogenates, these materials may make intimate contact and undergo metabolic reactions which bear no relation to those which actually occur *in vivo*.

The parasitological biochemist faces a further problem; for factors related to the presence of a different species, namely the host, are present *in vivo*. Thus, interactions between host and parasite metabolisms—such as, for example, the possible utilisation of each other's Krebs cycle intermediates—could occur, interactions which could not reasonably be predicted from *in vitro* results with homogenates of the parasite species alone.

Many (but not all) biochemists, admitting this limitation to the results obtained in their artificial systems, appreciate that such results produce only potential working hypotheses which must ultimately be tested with the intact, living system.

Nutrition

The term ' feeding ' is normally associated with an organism which possesses a mouth by which food is physically ingested. Organisms lacking ' mouths ', such as some protozoa or cestodes, are said to ' absorb ' semi- digested materials from the intestine, and it has long been assumed that cestodes lie in a bath of semi-digested ' soup ' from which they can extract nutriment, although the actual processes whereby this absorption is accomplished have been somewhat ignored. Tritiated thymidine or cytosine, for example, is rapidly incorporated into the nuclei of *H. microstoma* from a liquid medium.[97]

Evidence from metabolic and *in vitro* studies now suggests that a complex nutritional relationship occurs between a cestode and its host. Two surprising facts have emerged from such studies. The first is that cestodes, like plants and some microorganisms, are capable of ' fixing ' CO_2 (p. 76). This is clearly an efficient use of waste metabolic materials from the host intestinal mucosa. It is known that the mucosal cells have a high metabolic rate associated, no doubt, with the exceptionally high ' turnover time ' (p. 27), so that a high level of intestinal CO_2 can be expected; a level of 15% has been reported in the dog.[296]

The second unexpected finding is that some species at least, appear to be capable of taking in nutritional material by direct contact with the mucosal wall (p. 182). The evidence for this is based on *in vitro* studies with *Echinococcus granulosus*, which will only be outlined here but discussed in detail in Chapter 10. Briefly, it has been shown that the organism will develop *in vitro* in a strobilar direction only if it is provided with a solid, or semi-solid, proteinaceous substrate with which it can make intimate contact. In the absence of this substrate, a larval protoscolex reverts to growth in a cystic direction (Fig. 72). That the strobilar growth is not merely a matter of a contact-stimulus is shown from the fact that contact with a non-nutrient base, such as agar, does not result in strobilar growth (Fig. 75). This result is interpreted as demonstrating that the scolex of this cestode, which has a penetrative type of rostellum and normally embeds in a crypt of Lieberkühn, is in some way capable of directly absorbing materials from the mucosal surface. How this is done is not, as yet, known. It may be that the cestode tegument is merely ingesting particles of mucus or cellular debris by pinocytosis (p. 13). Alternatively, it may be that the scolex is actually secreting proteolytic or other enzymes, which attack the intestinal mucosa or the degenerating cells or mucus secretions released from it; membrane digestion (p. 90) may be involved (Fig. 76).

In vitro techniques are not sufficiently advanced to determine whether the same phenomenon occurs in other cestodes with a penetrative rostellum. If it does, our general ideas of how a cestode obtains its nutrition will require revision. The presence of glands in the scolex of many species (p. 17) may be a further indication of release of digestive enzymes at the point of attachment, although the enzymatic nature of these glands has not yet been demonstrated.

In the case of *H. nana*, although the extended rostellum penetrates into a crypt of Lieberkühn (Fig. 6), scolex contact with a nutritive substrate appears to be unnecessary for survival and growth, since this species will mature *in vitro* in a liquid medium *without* a solid substrate (p. 173).

Although sufficient evidence is not yet available to draw a firm conclusion, it may be found that cestodes fall into two groups; (*a*) those in which the scolex acts as an organ of nutrition as well as one of attachment (p. 182); (*b*) those in which the scolex acts simply as an organ of attachment.

A cestode which makes the maximum use of all avenues for obtaining nutrition can thus be envisaged as lying in the gut cavity with its strobila bathed in semi-digested, semi-solid food, from which it is absorbing food materials (by diffusion, active transport and possibly pinocytosis) through its tegument. Furthermore, the nutritive materials available from the intestine are supplemented (*a*) by carbon and oxygen atoms obtained from fixing CO_2 and (*b*) by materials released at the host-parasite interface, probably under the action of digestive enzymes (possibly membrane-bound), secreted by the scolex, and (*c*) by soluble constituents released or diffusing from the mucosal cells.

Chemical Composition

Quantitative Data

General comments. A considerable quantity of data has been accumulated on the chemical composition of cestodes[36]; the available information is summarised in Table 9. Although many of these data have been obtained as a result of the application of apparently precise chemical procedures, results must be interpreted with caution if they are to have any real significance. There are three reasons for this cautious approach. Firstly, many of the methods used, especially by earlier workers, may be open to criticism on technical grounds, and such methods would not be acceptable to modern workers. Secondly, there

TABLE 9

Chemical analysis of cestodes expressed as a percentage of the dry weight. For these figures to be of value the nutritional condition of the host at the time of autopsy should be known. Some of the figures may be based on methods of doubtful validity.

Figures in italics have been calculated from authors' data.

Species	Dry wt. as % of fresh wt.	Glycogen	Lipid	Protein	Inorganic substances	Stage	References
Anoplocephala magna (Taenia plicata)	27·5	6	33·1	—	1·22	adult	34
Calliobothrium verticillatum	27·6	—	—	—	—	adult	308
Cittotaenia perplexa	27·1	—	—	20·60	—	adult	52
Diphyllobothrium latum	—	17·9	—	—	—	plerocercoid	238
Diphyllobothrium latum	9·0	20	16·6	60	4·8	adult	34
Diphyllobothrium sp.	29·9	31·5	—	41	—	plerocercoid	13
Diphyllobothrium sp.	30·8	36·2	—	48	—	adult	13
Dipylidium caninum	20·4	—	—	—	—	adult	34
Echinococcus granulosus	14·8	19·8	13·6	62·5	13·5	protoscoleces	6
Eubothrium rugosum	—	22·8	—	—	—	adult	34
Hydatigera (Taenia) taeniaeformis	22·3	19·7	4·2	27·1	29·0	strobilocercus (mice)	38
Hydatigera (Taenia) taeniaeformis	28	43·3	5·3	26·3	18·1	strobilocercus (mice)	165, 169

						strobilocercus (rats)	38
Hydatigera (Taenia) taeniaeformis	29·5	24·9	3·1	28·9	28·4	strobilocercus (rats)	38
Hydatigera (Taenia) taeniaeformis	20	—	6·9	40·6	—	adult	165, 168
Hydatigera (Taenia) taeniaeformis	26·7	23·2	6·3	45·0	22·0	adult	38
* Hymenolepis diminuta	22·4	45·7	20·1	31·0	—	adult	101
Hymenolepis citelli	—	—	16·1	—	—	adult	143
Ligula intestinalis	29·0	38–52	—	35–45	—	plerocercoid	417
Moniezia expansa	9·2–11·0	24–32	30·1	21·8	10·5	adult	34, 36, 52
Multiceps multiceps (Coenurus cerebralis)	25·3	—	—	—	27·4	scolex	34
Multiceps multiceps	12·4	—	—	—	4·1	membranes	34
Raillietina cesticillus	20·5	22·4	15·5	36·4	11·5	adult	417
Schistocephalus solidus	31·8	50·9	—	35·8	5·8	plerocercoid	162
Schistocephalus solidus	38	28·0	—	—	—	adult	417
Taenia crassiceps	20	27·5	—	—	—	larva	452
Taenia hydatigena (marginata)	23·5	28	4·9	—	—	adult	34
Taenia saginata	12·2	48·8	11·2	32·0	5·3	adult	34, 235
Taenia solium	8·7	25·4	16·2	46	6·4	adult	34
Thysanosoma actinioides	16·3	—	—	29·0	—	adult	52
Triaenophorus nodulosus	—	13·8	—	—	—	adult	34

* See also Table 10.

is increasing evidence that the chemical composition may vary with the 'strain' of a particular species of cestode as well as the 'strain' of the host. Thirdly, the composition may fluctuate within quite wide limits, depending on (a) the time of the autopsy in relation to the feeding habits of the host, and (b) the state of maturity of the region of the worm analysed. Some of these questions are discussed more fully below.

Difficulties in analysis. It is beyond the scope of this book to discuss the technical problems of chemical analysis in detail, but attention may be drawn to a few special points; some of these problems as they relate to cestodes have been discussed by von Brand[35] and Hopkins.[165] For example, the majority of analyses of the glucose concentrations in cestodes have been carried out using the non-specific chemical methods, which are dependent on the reducing properties of sugars; these methods tend to give high values. It is claimed that an enzymatic method, using glucose oxidase, is considerably more accurate.[35] These considerations could explain the divergence in the glucose concentrations reported in *H. diminuta* as 80–380 mg per cent. by chemical methods and only 40 mg per cent. by the glucose oxidase method. Moreover, although only very low levels of trehalose occur in cestodes, the fact that workers relied on reducing methods prevented the identification of this carbohydrate in other platyhelminths.

The dry weight of cestode tissue may also be a source of error or confusion; this is of special importance, as other analytical figures are often quoted on a dry weight basis. Thus, in *Hydatigera taeniaeformis*, the water content of larvae up to eight months old is $72 \pm 3\%$, but in some older strobilocerci it rises to 80%. In adult worms the water content increases with age during the first eighteen days of infection and some variation occurs thereafter due to inter- and intra-host factors.[169] Hence the dry/fresh weight ratio will vary with age (Fig. 15).

'Strain' and chemical composition. There is increasing evidence (p. 4) that different 'strains' of the same 'species' of cestodes can occur, and therefore it is not surprising to find that such strains may differ biochemically. This may be related to a truly genetic variation in the cestode, but it may also be related to metabolic or nutritional differences in the strain of host utilised. These two factors are clearly interdependent to some extent, and may not be always separable. Thus, the glycogen content of *H. diminuta* obtained from one strain of rats (Long-Evans) was 32% (dry weight), whereas a figure of 63% (dry weight) was obtained from specimens from rats of a different strain (Sprague-Dawley).[302]

Host nutrition and chemical composition. The nutritional state of the host can have a profound influence on the chemical composition of cestodes.[417] The carbohydrate composition of cestodes is especially liable to fluctuate, and falls during periods of host starvation or rises during periods of host feeding. For example, the glycogen content of *Raillietina cesticillus* has been shown to fall from 4·6% (wet weight) to 0·25% during twenty hours of host starvation. Since the dry weight may be substantially affected by a change in carbohydrate content,

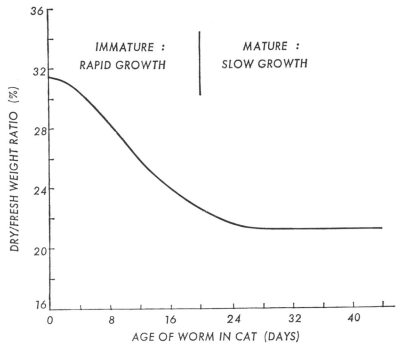

FIG. 15. The dry/fresh weight ratio of *Hydatigera taeniaeformis* developing in the intestine of a cat; scatter points omitted. (After Hopkins & Hutchison, 1960.)

the value of other constituents, such as protein, which are often expressed as a percentage of the dry weight, may not represent a reliable figure. Thus, in starved or 'bileless' rats, the carbohydrate content of *H. diminuta* has been shown to fall substantially, but this fall was accompanied by a rise in protein level.[125, 126]

The chemical composition may vary not only with the maturity of the region of worm analysed (Table 10) but also with the region of the intestine from which the worms are obtained. Thus, the protein content of *Diphyllobothrium* from the posterior one-third of the small intestine has been shown to be some 50% more than worms obtained from the anterior two-thirds (Fig. 16).

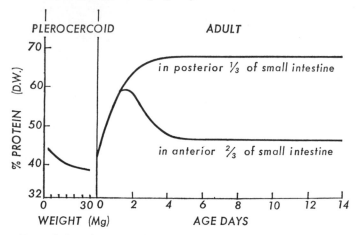

FIG. 16. Protein composition of *Diphyllobothrium* sp., expressed as a % of the dry weight. The % in the larva is plotted against fresh weight, that of the adult against age in the definitive host (rat); scatter points omitted. (Modified from Archer & Hopkins, 1958b.)

Composition of Major Constituents

Tissue composition. Cestodes are made up of the usual tissue constituents—protein, carbohydrates and lipids—but the proportions show a somewhat different pattern from that of most other invertebrates, in that the carbohydrate content tends to be unusually high and the protein, per unit of body weight, relatively low (Table 9). The nature of the protein and lipid constituents are discussed further in Chapter 6, but the high carbohydrate content is worthy of some special comment here.

In both larval and adult cestodes, the carbohydrate occurs mainly as glycogen—a polysaccharide which serves typically as one of the most important energy sources of helminths inhabiting biotopes with a low oxygen tension. Glycogens from various parasites show a high degree of polydispersity, i.e. they exhibit a broad spectrum of molecular weights. Moreover, this spectrum in *H. diminuta* (as determined by sedimentation coefficients) varies with the method of glycogen extraction used.[278]

Although the main carbohydrate of cestodes is referred to as ' glycogen ', the properties of cestode glycogens have not been well characterised, and some results obtained by the older analytical methods may have to be discounted.[36]   In *H. diminuta* and *R. cesticillus*, the glycogen is not found free but forms part of protein complexes.[191, 192]   In *Moniezia expansa*, the glycogen present has been shown to be similar to the glycogens of a number of vertebrate tissues with regard to the

TABLE 10

Chemical analyses of Hymenolepis diminuta *in different stages of maturity* (Data from Fairbairn, Wertheim, Harpur & Schiller[101])

Stages		Carbohydrates	Lipids	Nitrogen (as protein)
		(% Composition, dry weight basis)		
From 15-day-old worms	Immature proglottids	47	15	29
	Mature proglottids	46	18	26
	Pre-gravid and gravid proglottids	48	20	22
From 25-day-old worms	Infective proglottids (terminal 50 mm)	23	31	40
	Infective eggs	12	11	72

glucose residues per repeating unit (12 for *Moniezia*) and specific rotation (+194), although it cannot be assumed that the various glycogens in cestodes and vertebrates are identical.[316]

Larval cestodes are particularly rich in glycogen, which may reach quite astonishing levels—over 50% in the case of the plerocercoid larvae of pseudophyllideans, such as *Ligula* or *Diphyllobothrium* (Table 9).

Histochemical studies have shown that in cestodes glycogen occurs in expected tissue sites, namely the parenchyma and muscles (especially those of the suckers); the nervous, excretory and reproductive systems are generally free from glycogen.[65, 149, 200, 316, 490]

Calcareous corpuscles.   Many species of both trematodes and cestodes contain large numbers of curious concretions termed *calcareous corpuscles.*   These are especially noticeable in larval forms, and the numbers present vary widely even in the same species.   Calcareous corpuscles consist of an organic base together with inorganic material. They have been the subject of a number of studies.[42-5, 68, 375]

The organic material is reported to contain DNA, RNA, proteins, glycogen, a hyaluronic-type polysaccharide and alkaline phosphatase.[67, 68] The inorganic material consists mainly of Ca, Mg, P and CO_2 (Table 11), but traces of other metallic elements have been reported (Table 12). Although the levels of Ca, Mg and CO_2 show some uniformity, the quantity of phosphorus varies widely (Table 11).   In *Echinococcus granulosus*, the composition of the inorganic constituents also varies

TABLE 11

Composition of isolated, dried calcareous corpuscles in cestodes ; expressed as percentage of dried material
(Data from von Brand et al.[42, 43, 44])

Species	CaO	MgO	P_2O_5	CO_2
Cysticerus cellulosae	21·2	11·7	1·1	42·1
Cysticercus fasciolaris	24·9	22·2	4·0	31·9
Diphyllobothrium latum	13·0	23·8	29·7	18·0
Spirometra mansonoides	13·5	15·8	6·2	36·0
Echinococcus granulosus	20·5	13·8	2·7	32·0
Taenia hydatigena (marginata)	36·1	17·1	14·1	33·1
Taenia saginata	14·2	17·1	22·8	28·0
Hydatigera taeniaeformis	28·0	17·4	11·3	27·9

slightly in specimens from different countries (Table 12). This may perhaps reflect minor ' strain ' differences in this species (p. 5). Electron microscope studies show that calcareous corpuscles are formed within cells and are composed of concentric lamellae.[42, 375] The mineral content of these bodies is amorphous but can be converted to a crystalline form by heating (Plate II).

TABLE 12

Minor components of the calcareous corpuscles of Echinococcus granulosus *as determined by emission spectroscopic analysis (Melpar)*
(Data from von Brand, et al.[43])

	Material from		
	Chile	New Zealand	Lebanon
Aluminium	+	+	+
Boron	—	—	—
Cadmium	+	+	+
Copper	—	—	—
Iron	+	+	+
Lead	—	—	—
Manganese	—	+	+
Nickel	+	+	+
Sodium	+	+	+
Strontium	+	+	+
Tin	—	—	—
Titanium	+	+	+

The function of calcareous corpuscles is not known. In *H. taeniae-formis*, corpuscle material disappears more rapidly in the absence than in the presence of oxygen; the material is also lost in acid but not in alkaline media. This has led to the suggestion that one function of the calcareous corpuscles could be to buffer anaerobically produced acids.[42] It is probable, however, that the role of the corpuscles is more complex than this, and the high level of inorganic ions leads to the speculation

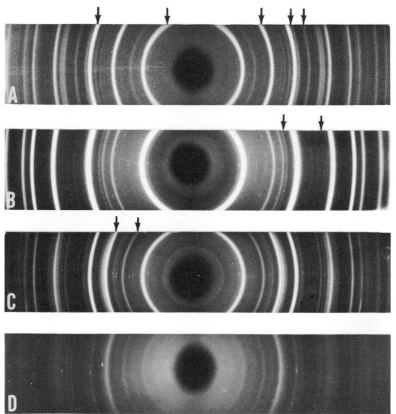

PLATE II. Diffraction patterns in calcareous corpuscles of cestodes. A. *Cysticercus cellulosae*—brucite (left arrows), calcite (right arrows). B. *Spirometra mansonoides*—brucite, traces of calcite, $Ca(OH)_2$ (arrows). C. *Taenia saginata*—brucite, hydroxyapatite (arrows), $Ca(OH)_2$. D. *Diphyllobothrium latum*—brucite, hydroxyapatite. (After von Brand, Scott, Nylen & Pugh, 1965.)

that corpuscles may act as major reserve centres for such ions. Thus, when a larva enters the intestine of a host, it is faced with a metabolic situation in which a large amount of energy is immediately required for (a) muscular activity for attachment, (b) rapid initial growth, and (c) the active transport of nutritive materials. Clearly, the calcareous corpuscles could provide CO_2 (without the necessity of its being transported through the tegument from exogenous sources), which would then be available for fixation (p. 76), in addition to Mg^{2+} ions, which are well known to catalyse several reactions in the Embden-Meyerhof glycolysis pathway p. 71), and phosphate, which is used in phosphorylating reactions. A possible confirmation of this view is the fact that the first indication of strobilar development of *Echinococcus* is a gradual but observable, reduction in the numbers of the calcareous corpuscles, which finally disappear completely.[423, 473] In this species, the corpuscles reappear when the third proglottid develops.

Further confirmation that the corpuscles may act as a reservoir of phosphate come from experiments with ^{32}P, on *H. taeniaeformis*.[45] Thus, it has been shown that *in vitro* and *in vivo* larval *H. taeniaeformis* rapidly accumulates ^{32}P both in its tissues and its calcareous corpuscles. The uptake, which appears to be by diffusion and not by active transport (p. 30), is influenced by Na^+ and CO_3; lowering the temperature has very little effect (Table 13). The absorbed phosphate becomes tightly bound to the corpuscles and cannot be removed by washing.

TABLE 13

Incorporation of inorganic orthophosphate ($^{32}P_i$) into isolated calcareous corpuscles of Hydatigera taeniaeformis
(Data from von Brand & Weinbach[45])

Time (min.)	37°		6°	
	Radioactivity (c.p.m./mg dry wt.)	P_i uptake (μ moles)	Radioactivity (c.p.m./mg dry wt.)	P_i uptake (μ moles)
0	$3\cdot1 \times 10^3$	2·3	$2\cdot5 \times 10^3$	2·6
5	5·0	5·0	3·6	4·2
10	5·9	5·2	4·6	4·4
15	5·3	5·1	4·5	4·8
60	6·5	6·5	6·3	5·9
120	8·2	7·6	6·2	6·3

Respiration

General Considerations

Consideration of the oxygen consumption of cestodes raises a number of questions of great physiological interest, many of which are at present unsolved. Two general conclusions can be drawn.

(a) Under experimental conditions, all species of cestodes so far examined have been found to utilise oxygen when it is available; (b) fermentation* persists at almost the same rate under complete anaerobiosis as under atmospheric oxygen tension (Table 19).[37]

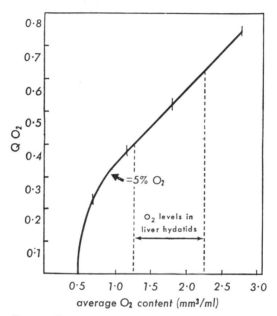

FIG. 17. Oxygen consumption of *Echinococcus granulosus* in hydatid fluid, as a function of oxygen tension of the fluid. (From Read & Simmons, 1963, after Farhan, *et al.*, 1959.)

In relation to the figures obtained for oxygen consumption (Table 14) it must be emphasised that results obtained in (say) a Warburg respirometer under a gas phase of air, are of uncertain value, since it is unlikely that *in vivo* a parasite has access to an oxygen tension of this order. Moreover, experimental determinations *in vitro* are very dependent on such factors as the incubation medium used, the age and condition of the cestode tissue, and, sometimes, the host from which the material was obtained. In a detailed study of respiration of adult and larval *H. taeniaeformis*,[38] it was found that larvae from rats had a

---

* ' Fermentation ' is a somewhat unsatisfactory term for which there seems to be no adequate substitute. Originally used to denote the ability of organisms to utilise glucose in the absence of oxygen, it was later realised that aerobic cells can perform ' fermentations '.

higher Q_{O_2} than those from mice; also larvae (from rats) respired at a higher rate when incubated in serum than when incubated in Tyrode (Table 14).

To obtain meaningful figures for respiration, it is necessary, therefore, to know the oxygen tension at the precise site of establishment of the parasite and to determine the oxygen consumption of the cestode at this tension. The likely oxygen level of the alimentary canal has already been discussed (Chapter 3); it appears to be low in the lumen, higher in the liquid in contact with the mucosa and, probably, higher still within the crypts of Lieberkühn.

The fact that *H. nana* can be cultured to maturity *in vitro*[393] in a gas phase of 5% CO_2 in N_2 indicates that some species can develop in an entirely anaerobic environment, whereas others (e.g. *Echinococcus granulosus*), which penetrate more deeply into the mucosa, require oxygen for normal strobilar development *in vitro*.[430] The oxygen consumption of *Echinococcus* ceases entirely below about 5% O_2 (representing an O_2 tension of 0·8 mm³/ml[102] (Fig. 17); but above this tension the organism is a conformer, i.e. its metabolic rate is adjusted to the amount of oxygen available in the environment.

In *H. diminuta* too, the oxygen consumption is markedly dependent on oxygen tension and, as in *Echinococcus*, falls sharply at a tension of about 5% O_2 (Fig. 18). In *H. diminuta* the endogenous *R.Q.* average is 0·51 and, in the presence of glucose, 1·02.[302] This suggests that this species oxidises glucose to CO_2 and H_2O. However, even if all the O_2 utilised is involved in glucose oxidation, it still accounts for less than 5% of the glucose removed from the medium.

In *Diphyllobothrium*, at a tension of 5% O_2, anterior and posterior proglottids take up 91% and 66% respectively of the rate at 21% O_2.[108] It must be remembered that this species, being a pseudophyllidean, forms a quinone-tanned egg, so that some of the O_2 may have been utilised for the process of egg-shell formation and tanning (p. 112), which involves phenolases (*o*-diphenol: O_2 oxidoreductase). The higher Q_{O_2} in the anterior proglottids may reflect the higher requirements of the active differentiation taking place in that region.

In *Schistocephalus solidus* the Q_{O_2} displays thermal acclimation on a seasonal basis, and is higher in winter than in summer. The Q_{10} in this species decreases at temperatures up to 30°C, but then increases at temperatures from 30 to 40°C, suggesting that at higher temperatures alternative enzyme pathways are used (p. 157).[92]

Respiration and Size

The relationship between metabolic rate and size is usually studied by measuring the rate of O_2 consumption and has been investigated in many homeothermic and poikilothermic animals. This question is complicated in cestodes, since (*a*) there is no definite end-point in cestode growth and (*b*) an adult cestode—unlike most organisms which have a specific degree of tissue differentiation related to size—consists of a series of stages of embryonic differentiation ranging from undifferen-

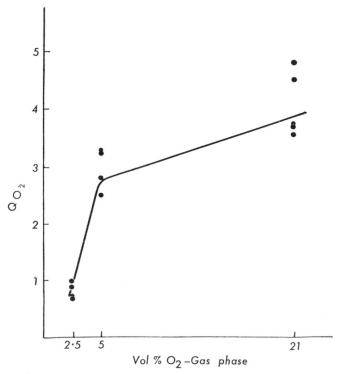

FIG. 18. Effect of varying oxygen tension on the oxygen consumption of *Hymenolepis diminuta*. (After Read, 1956.)

tiated tissue (immediately posterior to the scolex) to the fully differentiated and mature tissues in the posterior proglottids. It is not surprising therefore, to find that cestodes do not fall neatly into the characteristic metabolic rate/size relationships presented by other invertebrate groups.[37]

The relationship between body weight and metabolic rate in cestodes can be expressed[37, 92] as

$$Y = \hat{a}X^b$$

TABLE 14

O_2 consumption of some cestodes in atmospheric air; additional figures of earlier workers are given by von Brand[34]

Species	Stage	Temp. °C.	Incubation medium	Q_{O_2} (μl. O_2/mg. dry wt./hr.)		References
				sugar absent	sugar present	
Diphyllobothrium latum	plerocercoid	24	0·9% NaCl	0·55	0·78	108
Diphyllobothrium latum	proglottids—mature	37	Ringer	2·36	—	108
Schistocephalus solidus	plerocercoid (winter)	30	Tyrode	0·48	—	92
Schistocephalus solidus	plerocercoid (summer)	30	Tyrode	0·33	—	92
Moniezia expansa	scolex	37	Ringer	—	1·1	11
Moniezia expansa	proglottids—mature	37	Ringer	—	0·9	11
Moniezia expansa	proglottids—gravid	37	Ringer	—	0·6	11
Hymenolepis diminuta	adult	37	Krebs-Ringer	1·2	3·0	302
Taenia crassiceps	larva	37	Hank's?	1·3	1·3	452
Hydatigera taeniaeformis	strobilocercus (mice)	37	cat serum	0·53	—	38
Hydatigera taeniaeformis	strobilocercus (rat)	37	cat serum	0·64	—	38
Hydatigera taeniaeformis	strobilocercus (rat)	37	Tyrode	0·47	—	38
Hydatigera taeniaeformis	adult	37	Tyrode	1·15	—	38
Echinococcus granulosus	protoscoleces	37	Ringer	1·8	—	6
Echinococcus granulosus	protoscoleces	37	hydatid fluid	0·85	—	102
Echinococcus granulosus	protoscoleces	37	Parker 199*	—	1·7	421

* + Amniotic fluid.

where Y = volume of O_2 consumed (aerobic metabolism) or CO_2 produced (anaerobic metabolism) in unit time; X = body weight; $\hat{a}$, $\hat{b}$ = constants.

Taking logarithms of each side of the above equation,

$$\log Y = \log \hat{a} + \hat{b} \log X,$$

we obtain a straight-line relationship.

Now, if cestodes are considered as long, flattened cylinders, it follows that their surface area is roughly proportional to their weight.[37] If the rate of gaseous exchange were related directly to the surface area (i.e. to the weight) the value of $\hat{b}$ would be 1·0. In fact in *H. taeniaeformis* the value of $\hat{b}$ lies between 0·5 and 1·0, so that clearly in this species O_2 consumption is not related directly to either body weight or surface area. A comparable position has been found in *Schistocephalus* where the $\hat{b}$ values lie between −0·087 and −0·639; nor does the temperature at which respiration is measured (10–40°C) influence these figures.[92] This result is not surprising since, as will be discussed below, it is unlikely that O_2 consumed by cestodes is utilised entirely in the same way as by animals with a completely aerobic type of metabolism.[37] Both trematodes and nematodes are known to have largely anaerobic metabolisms, even at atmospheric oxygen tensions.[215a, 422]

Significance of Oxygen Consumption

It is difficult, with the data available, to deduce the significance of oxygen consumption in the metabolism of cestodes. It has been conjectured[302] that oxygen may play a more important part in the production of intermediate compounds of value in metabolism than in the production of energy; clearly in some species both these processes are likely to be occurring in parallel. Since cestodes have neither a circulatory system nor a respiratory pigment, the oxygen tension within the strobila will be determined by the external oxygen tension and the diffusion coefficient of the tissues.[302] If O_2 is utilised by tissues, a concentration gradient from the peripheral to the central tissues will result; the tension in the central region may thus be zero. If by-products of the central anaerobic metabolism could diffuse to the peripheral tissue, they could be oxidised there; conversely, peripherally oxidised products could be available, after diffusion, in the centre.[302]

The terminal oxidation processes are discussed later (p. 82).

5: The Adult: Carbohydrate Metabolism

General Account

General Comments

The carbohydrate metabolism of cestodes has been more intensively studied than any other aspect of metabolism; it has been the subject of a number of reviews.[34, 35, 36, 305-6, 316, 417] The main questions to be answered when discussing carbohydrate metabolism are: (*a*) what carbohydrates are utilised exogenously? (*b*) by what mechanisms are they absorbed, and (*c*) what metabolic pathways are followed?

Although much work has been done on these problems, many results reported may be open to criticism on the technical grounds that the conditions under which the experiments were carried out were not sufficiently close to those occurring *in vivo*. For example, it is known that CO_2 is a constituent of the intestinal gases (p. 35), and it has been shown that the presence or absence of CO_2 *in vitro* can have a profound effect on the uptake of glucose in *H. diminuta*.[101, 307] Thus, in the presence of CO_2 the synthesis of glycogen and utilisation of glucose were found to be 7–8 times more effective than when CO_2 was lacking (Table·15). This effect is chiefly related to CO_2-fixation and the

TABLE 15

Carbohydrate metabolism of Hymenolepis diminuta *in the presence and absence of* CO_2.
(Data from Fairbairn, *et al.*[101])

Treatment	Carbohydrate synthesised	Glucose utilised	Glucose fermented	Acids excreted	Succinic acid excreted
	(g per 3·97 g fresh wt. worms)				
Krebs-Ringer-glucose (gas phase 5% CO_2; 95% N_2)	0·184	0·360	0·176	3·19	2·26
Krebs-Ringer-phosphate glucose (gas phase N_2)	0·020	0·049	0·029	0·58	0·31

57

utilisation of the fumarate formed to reoxidise the NADH formed during glycolysis (p. 77).[101] The pattern of excretory products was also markedly different under the two conditions. This important result suggests that earlier work carried out on the absorption of exogenous carbohydrate in the absence of CO_2 will undoubtedly require re-evaluation.

Polysaccharides other than Glycogen

The occurrence and the distribution of glycogen in cestodes have been dealt with in the previous chapter. Although glycogen is the main polysaccharide in cestode tissues, several others have been reported.

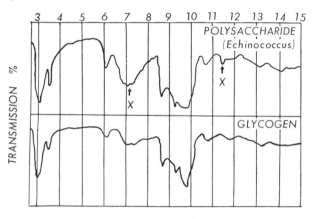

WAVELENGTH   (microns)

FIG. 19. Infra-red spectra of polysaccharide isolated from protoscoleces of *Echinococcus granulosus* by Pflüger's method, compared with the spectrum of commercial glycogen. X=bands due to unknown contaminant. (Kilejian, *et al.*, 1962.)

In *E. granulosus*, a polysaccharide with a base of glucosamine, galactose and/or glucose was isolated from the laminated membrane of the hydatid cyst, the protoscoleces and the cyst fluid.[73, 77, 199] A polysaccharide extract, obtained by Pflüger's method, had an infra-red spectrum (Fig. 19) comparable to that of a commercial sample of glycogen.[199] When polysaccharide was isolated by an alternative method (Gary's) a different spectrum was obtained (Fig. 20), indicating the presence of another polysaccharide, which was destroyed by Pflüger's method. This proved to be a mucopolysaccharide or polysaccharide-protein complex. This result further emphasises the point, made earlier (p. 46), that different analytical methods may give different

results.   This new material had absorption bands in the region of
$8·5\,\mu$ to $10·0\,\mu$, strongly indicative of a polysaccharide; but, in addition,
bands occurred at $6·1\,\mu$, and $6·5\,\mu$—regions usually indicative of protein.
More detailed work indicated the presence of a galactosamine, and also
pointed to the likelihood of a protein-carbohydrate complex in
Echinococcus.[205]

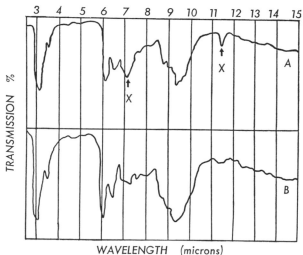

FIG. 20. Infra-red spectra of mucopolysaccharide isolated
from scoleces of *Echinococcus granulosus* by (A) Gary's
method, after acetone precipitation, (B) Gary's method,
after glycogen removal and alcohol precipitation.   Both
spectra are almost identical, except for an unknown
contaminant, X, at $7·1\mu$ and $11·4\mu$. (After Kilejian *et al*,
1962.)

The occurrence of mucopolysaccharide is of especial interest, because
an antigenic polysaccharide extracted from the cyst membranes of *E.
granulosus* has previously been reported.[73]   An antigenic mucopolysaccharide, which appears to be antigenically identical with the human
P blood group substance, has also been detected by the fluorescent antibody technique.[431]   These antigens may prove to be one and the same
substance.   The immunological significance of these results is discussed
further in Chapter 12.

Utilisation of Exogenous Carbohydrate

In vivo *Experiments*

Cestodes have substantial carbohydrate requirements, and for their
normal development and reproduction carbohydrate must be present

in the host diet (contrast proteins, p. 61). Thus, when a rat infected with *H. diminuta* is placed on a diet devoid of carbohydrate, there is a marked decrease in the size and number of strobila.[305] Over a critical range of 0·1–3·0 gm starch per day, the strobila size and rate of reproduction attained by *H. diminuta* appear to be linear functions of the absolute quantity of carbohydrate taken daily by the host.[315] Differences between species and the strain of host are also important in considering metabolism. The two related species, *H. citelli* and *H. nana*, for instance, require the inclusion of carbohydrate in the host diet; but

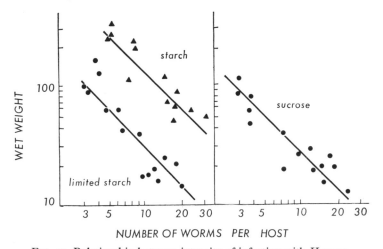

FIG. 21. Relationship between intensity of infection with *Hymeno-lepis diminuta* and mean weight of individual worms in rats fed on (a) unlimited starch, (b) limited starch (1·0 g. per day) and (c) sucrose. Standard error bars omitted. (Modified from Read & Phifer, 1959.)

the growth of *H. nana*, is affected only if carbohydrate is not available during the early period of establishment.[305] Experiments establishing the relationship between starch in the diet and worm growth have been criticised on the grounds that the calorific intake also varies with increased starch intake. However, when the carbohydrate content was varied isocalorically (i.e. by adjusting other diet constituents) comparable results were obtained.[240]

These differences emphasise the importance of understanding the life cycle and developmental pattern of a species of cestode when attempting to interpret biochemical results. There are, for example, important differences between the developmental history of *H. diminuta* and that of *H. nana*. *H. diminuta* grows at a more or less constant rate throughout its adult life, i.e. it shows no evidence of senescence.   In contrast, growth of *H. nana* is rapid for only 10–12 days after reaching the intestine and thereafter new segments are produced more slowly; carbohydrate requirements, therefore, would be high only during the early phases of establishment and strobilar differentiation.   *H. citelli* appears to be intermediate between *H. nana* and *H. diminuta* both in its growth characteristics and in its response to carbohydrate deficiency.[315]   Similar work on *Raillietina* in birds,[324] *Oochoristica* in rodents[303] and *Lacistorhynchus* in dogfish,[303] confirms that carbohydrate in the host diet is a necessity for cestode growth.

The quality of host carbohydrate also has an effect on growth, as does the level of infection in a host, i.e. there is a ' crowding ' effect (p. 159) related to the number of worms present.   In host rats fed on (*a*) starch *ad lib.*, (*b*) limited starch, or (*c*) sucrose, the size of worm decreased in proportion as the worm burden increased in all three cases (Fig. 21).[309]   One of the most interesting results found when examining the effect of the host diet on cestode growth was that worms grew *better* in a host fed on a protein-free diet containing carbohydrate (Table 16) than in one containing both carbohydrate and protein.[240] The explanation of this unexpected finding is probably related to the fact that the amino acid levels in the intestine remain relatively high —due partly to a ' leak back ' from the intestinal wall into the lumen (p. 28).

In vitro *Experiments*

Type of carbohydrate utilised.   A substantial amount of experimental work has been carried out on the utilisation of exogenous carbohydrate during short periods of maintenance *in vitro*.   As we emphasised earlier, some of this work may need re-evaluation because of unsuitability of the physiological conditions under which the experiments were carried out.   Attention has already been drawn (Table 15) to the fact that the uptake of glucose by *H. diminuta* is more effective when CO_2 is present than when it is absent.

The presence of Na^+ ions too, has a marked influence on glucose uptake and, in their absence, *H. taeniaeformis* fails to take up glucose.[40]

The available data on the utilisation of exogenous carbohydrates *in vitro* are summarised in Table 17.   All species examined utilised glucose, and most of them used galactose; but maltose was utilised by only three species, and sucrose by one.   Only in *Cittotaenia* sp.,[313] and *Phyllobothrium foliatum*[214] was maltose metabolised at a higher rate than glucose.   The mechanism of uptake of carbohydrate is not known, but the evidence (p. 63) indicating that this takes place by active transport, as in vertebrate intestinal cells, is now impressive.[41, 286–8, 305]

TABLE 16

Effect of substituting fat or carbohydrate for dietary protein on the weight and nitrogen content of Hymenolepis diminuta in rats
(Data from Mettrick & Munro[240])

Host Diet	Host				Parasite			
	Initial body wt. (g.)	Body wt. change (g.)	Liver wt. (g.)	Liver protein N/100 g. body wt. (mg.)	Mean no. of worms/ rat	Dry wt./worm (mg.)	N/worm (mg.)	Non-protein dry wt./ worm (mg.)
Casein + normal carbohydrate	128	−5	4·7	109	11·0	29	2·0	17
Protein-free (fat-rich)	127	−22	4·0	79	9·0	34(+17%)	2·2(+10%)	20(+18%)
Protein-free (carbohydrate-rich)	129	−24	4·3	78	9·0	48(+66%)	3·0(+50%)	29(+71%)
Statistical significance of dietary effect	—	P<0·005	—	P<0·005	—	P<0·01	P<0·05	P<0·01

Utilisation of a carbohydrate, such as glucose, is complicated by the fact that a leakage of glucose and certain unidentified sugars has been demonstrated in *Hydatigera* (*Taenia*) *taeniaeformis* maintained in glucose-free saline; whereas distinctly less carbohydrate was lost by worms maintained in serum. The presence of galactose, mannose and fructose in the medium did not prevent, but could modify, the leakage of glucose. There is no evidence, however, that a glucose leakage can occur against a concentration gradient. An interesting result is that in Na^+-free or Na^+-poor Tyrode, the glucose leakage was greatly increased.[41] The precise significance of the glucose leakage is not clear.

In media containing glucose, glycogenesis is stimulated in many species, as is evidenced by a build-up of glycogen in the parenchyma.[41, 48, 101, 214, 301] In adult *H. taeniaeformis*, the glucose consumption has been reported to be independent of the external glucose concentration over a range of 12·5–200 mg per cent. initial concentration. In contrast, in larval *H. taeniaeformis* a transition from glucose leakage to glucose consumption occurs only when the external concentration reaches a level of 100–200 mg per cent.

A possible explanation of this difference[41], may lie in the fact that larvae—in contrast to adults in the gut where the carbohydrate levels may fluctuate widely—may have access to glucose at a more or less constant level in the liver of the rodent host. Absorption from low levels of glucose may not be necessary for survival in this case. The fate of absorbed glucose is not clear; there is no evidence to indicate what proportion is utilised directly for energy purposes via the Embden-Meyerhof pathway, or what proportion is utilised for glycogen synthesis and subsequently broken down to glucose. In *H. taeniaeformis*, ' free ' glucose can be detected in the worm tissues on incubation in glucose-containing media. In this species, there is no unequivocal evidence of polysaccharide synthesis, but rather there is evidence of a sparing of endogenous polysaccharide utilisation.

Evidence for active transport of carbohydrate. There is now convincing evidence that the movement of glucose, and presumably other carbohydrates, into cestodes cannot be accounted for in terms of simple diffusion, but takes place largely by active transport (p. 102). Much of the evidence for active transport has been based on *in vitro* experiments with *H. diminuta*.[41, 305, 316] Especially convincing have been the experiments of Phifer, using ^{14}C-labelled glucose.[286–288]

If entry of glucose into *H. diminuta* was merely a matter of simple diffusion, the rate of diffusion should be directly proportional to the concentration of glucose in the incubation medium. However, it was found that absorption of glucose by *H. diminuta* was independent of

TABLE 17

Exogenous carbohydrates utilised by cestodes in vitro.

(+++ to + levels of utilisation ; — not utilised ; · no information)

Species	* gas phase (where stated)	Glucose	Galactose	Mannose	Fructose	Xylose	Maltose	Sucrose	Lactose	Trehalose	Arabinose	Glucosamine	Refs.
Order CYCLOPHYLLIDEA													
Hymenolepis diminuta	5% CO_2	+++	++	+?	—	+?	—	—	—	—	—	—	213
Hymenolepis nana	5% CO_2	+++	++	—	—	·	—	—	—	—	·	·	313
Hymenolepis citelli	5% CO_2	+++	++	—	—	·	—	—	—	—	·	·	313
Oochoristica symmetrica	5% CO_2	+++	+++	+?	·	·	·	·	·	·	·	·	213
Cittotaenia sp.	5% CO_2	++	+	—	—	+++	+++	+++	—	—	·	·	313
Mesocestoides latus	5% CO_2	++	++	—	—	+	—	—	—	—	·	·	313
Moniezia expansa	?	+++	—	?	—	?	—	?	·	·	·	·	34
Hydatigera taeniaeformis (larvae)	5% CO_2	+++	+++	+	+?	·	·	·	·	·	·	·	41
Hydatigera taeniaeformis (adults)	5% CO_2	+++	+++	?	—	·	·	·	·	·	·	·	41
Echinococcus granulosus (protoscoleces)	N_2	+++	·	·	·	·	·	·	·	·	·	·	7
Echinococcus granulosus (adults)	5% CO_2 +10% O_2	+++	·	·	·	·	·	·	·	·	·	·	47
Taenia crassiceps	Air	+++	·	·	·	·	·	·	·	·	·	·	452

Order TRYPANORHYNCHA

Species														Refs
Lacistorhynchus tenuis	5% CO$_2$	+++	++	+	-	·	+	—	·	—	—	·	·	303, 214

Order TETRAPHYLLIDEA

Species														Refs
Onchobothrium pseudo-uncinatum	?	++	++	-	—	·	—	·	·	·	·	·	·	214
Phyllobothrium foliatum	?	+	+	-	—	—	+	·	·	·	·	·	·	214
Anthobothrium variable	?	+++	++	·	·	·	·	·	·	·	·	·	·	214
Inermiphyllidium pulvinatum	?	+++	++	-	·	+	·	·	·	·	·	·	·	214
Orygmatobothrium dohrnii	?	++	++	·	·	·	·	·	·	·	·	·	·	214
Disculiceps pileatum	?	+	+	+?	+?	·	-	·	·	·	·	·	·	214
Calliobothrium verticillatum	5% CO$_2$	+++	++	+?	+?	·	-	—	·	·	—	·	·	303

Order PSEUDOPHYLLIDEA

Species														Refs
Diphyllobothrium latum**	Air?	++++	·	·	·	·	·	·	·	·	·	·	·	34
Ligula intestinalis**	Air?	++++	·	·	·	·	·	·	·	·	·	·	·	34
Eubothrium rugosum	Air?	++++	·	·	·	·	·	·	·	·	·	·	·	34
Triaenophorus nodulosus	Air?	++++	·	·	·	·	·	·	·	·	·	·	·	34
Schistocephalus solidus	Air?	++++	·	·	·	·	·	·	·	·	·	·	·	34, 163

* in N$_2$ unless stated.

** plerocercoids.

the concentration once outside the limiting concentration (Fig. 22).[286, 307] Beyond about $1 \cdot 1 \times 10^{-2}$M, increasing the concentration of glucose did not result in an increase in the rate of absorption.[286] Furthermore, it was shown that metabolic inhibitors, such as para-chloromercuri-benzoate (PCMB) or 2,-4–dinitrophenol (DNP), greatly reduced uptake of glucose.[286]

Again, if absorption were a simple diffusion process, uptake of glucose should not theoretically be affected by pH. In *H. diminuta*, the uptake of glucose, measured over a period of 30 mins. showed a major peak at pH 7·5 with a minor peak at 8·5 (Fig. 23). These results suggest the probability that at least one enzyme system, and possibly two, are involved in the transport mechanism.

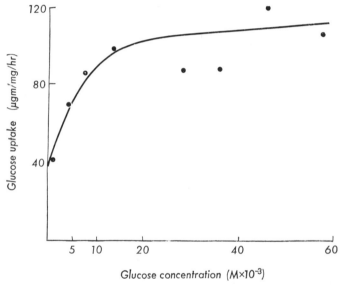

FIG. 22. Effect of glucose concentration on its uptake by *Hymeno-lepis diminuta* at pH 7·5 in 30 minutes. Optimum absorption occurs at 11×10^{-3}M. (After Phifer, 1960a.)

In considering this result, it will be recalled that alkaline phosphatase has been reported in the tegument of numerous species of cestodes (Table 2). Although a functional relationship between alkaline phosphatase and glucose transport has never been unequivocally demonstrated, the fact that it is present at high concentrations in vertebrate tissues sites such as the intestinal mucosa and proximal renal tubules—where active transport of glucose is known to occur—lends some theoretical support to this view. However, the whole question of the functions of acid and alkaline phosphatases is still very much unsolved.

It is of interest to note that both enzymes are also present in the trematode tegument across which glucose can similarly be absorbed.[422]

The fact that glucose absorption by cestodes is inhibited by the drug phlorizin is sometimes quoted as being further evidence that phosphatase is involved.   However, the drug inhibits glucose absorption in *H. diminuta* at a much lower concentration than is required to inhibit alkaline phosphatase.[286]   Moreover, $6 \cdot 5 \times 10^{-5}$ ammonium molybdate has been shown to inhibit the alkaline phosphatase of

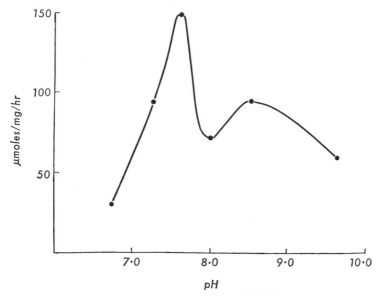

FIG. 23. Effect of *p*H on the rate of glucose uptake by *Hymenolepis diminuta*. (Glucose concentration, $8 \cdot 3 \times 10^{-3}$M; incubation time 30 minutes.) (After Phifer, 1960a.)

H. diminuta; yet this had no effect on the uptake of glucose by the worm, thus demonstrating that alkaline phosphatase activity was not directly involved in this process.[288]

Further evidence in favour of active transport of glucose is seen in the fact that in *H. diminuta* the uptake is accelerated on the twelfth day after infection, i.e. at a time when tissue differentiation is probably proceeding at a maximum rate.[286]   Since this difference can be shown to be unrelated to a size difference, it again suggests that a enzymatic process is involved.

The advantages to a cestode of utilising an active process for carbohydrate absorption, rather than merely relying on simple diffusion, are several.[287] Thus, should the glucose concentration in the gut fall to a low level, glucose uptake would not be possible if diffusion were the only means of transport, and indeed, some glucose might 'leak' out. Again, at very low concentrations, (even though higher than in the worm) the rate of diffusion might not be sufficient to satisfy the metabolic demands of the worm, especially as the tegument of the worm must operate in competition with the mucosal cells of the intestine.

TABLE 18

Quantitative details of carbohydrate metabolism of protoscoleces of Echinococcus granulosus
(Data from Agosin[1])

	Aerobiosis		Anaerobiosis	
	μ moles/grm. wet wt/3 hr.	Molar ratio	μ moles/grm. wet wt/3 hr.	Molar ratio
Glycogen consumed	11·97±2·50	1·00	13·50±1·6	1·00
Production of CO_2	—	—	18·33±0·76	1·322±0·06
O_2 Consumption	31·20±1·05	2·64±0·16	—	—
Pyruvic acid	0·91±0·28	0·063±0·03	0·0	—
Acetic acid	2·56±0·09	0·212±0·02	2·87±0·90	0·213±0·06
Succinic acid	1·19±0·20	0·099±0·01	7·0±0·90	0·517±0·74
Lactic acid	12·19±1·26	1·165±0·01	13·15±1·95	0·965±0·17
Ethyl alcohol	0·49±0·05	0·038±0·001	0·33±0·11	0·026±0·09

End-products of Carbohydrate Metabolism

In predominantly aerobic organisms, such as most free-living metazoa, the end-product of glycolysis is almost exclusively lactic acid from pyruvic acid (Table 20). This is produced as a result of rapid muscle contractions carried out essentially under anaerobic conditions. This mechanism enables a rapid expenditure of energy to occur by avoiding the limitation due to the rate of diffusion of oxygen.

The anaerobic phase is then followed normally by an aerobic phase in which much of the pyruvic acid undergoes oxidative decarboxylation to acetyl coenzyme A—and is oxidised further in the Krebs cycle (Table 21) to CO_2 and H_2O. If oxygen does not become available immediately after the anaerobic phase, an 'oxygen debt' is said to be built up. In cestodes, however, in common with trematodes[422] the lactic acid is not further metabolised—at least under *in vitro* conditions —but is secreted together with other fatty acids. It is not known if this represents the true *in vivo* situation.

Cestodes possess a high rate of fermentative metabolism, and lactic and succinic acids are the acids most generally excreted (Tables 18, 19). There is, however, considerable difference between species, and sometimes between adult and larva of the same species. The conditions under which a worm is maintained whilst its excretory products are being studied are of the utmost importance and may have a profound effect on the nature and quantities of the end-products produced. The gas phase, especially the pCO_2 and pO_2, is of especial importance, differences being reported, for example, between excretory products released by several species under anaerobic and aerobic conditions (Table 18). Unfortunately, not all authors have stated the

TABLE 19

Carbon balances in the metabolism of adult and larval Hydatigera taeniaeformis
(Data from von Brand & Bowman[38])

	Cysticercus fasciolaris				Adult *H. taeniaeformis*	
	From mice	From rats		From rats	From cats	
	In serum			In sugar-free Tyrode's	In sugar-free Tyrode's	
	Aerobic	Anaerobic	Aerobic	Anaerobic	Aerobic	Anaerobic
	%	%	%	%	%	%
Carbohydrate reserve of body	88	58	100	100	100	100
Absorbed from medium	12	42	—	—	—	—
Total carbohydrate utilised	100	100	100	100	100	100
Carbohydrate excreted	—	—	23	10	10	2
Carbohydrate potentially oxidised	11	13	5	—	17	—
Lactic acid	23	45	29	27	23	15
Pyruvic acid	3	3	3	1	3	1
Acetic acid	10	14	7	9	28	13
Succinic acid	—	2	2	25	22	48
Glycerol	1	4	1	2	1	1
Ethanol	9	12	< 1	< 1	1	1
Total carbon of metabolites	57	93	70	74	105	81

gas phase under which their experiments were carried out; this makes their results, if not actually invalid, at least open to question. The level of glucose is also significant and in *H. diminuta* an increase of up to six-fold in the acid production in the presence of glucose has been reported.[101]

With a few minor exceptions, almost all studies of end-products have been carried out on species of Cyclophyllidea, and only three species, *H. diminuta*, *Hydatigera taeniaeformis* and *E. granulosus* have been examined in any detail.   *H. taeniaeformis* excretes lactic, pyruvic, acetic and succinic acids, as well as ethanol.[38] Under anaerobic conditions the production of lactic acid decreased slightly, but much more succinic acid was produced.   The adult of this species also produced much greater amounts of succinate than the larva (*Cysticercus fasciolaris*) —a result at present not explained.

The position in *H. diminuta* is not clear, as different workers have given conflicting evidence.   Thus, lactic acid was reported[213] to account for 37–98% of the acid excreted.   In other experiments with the same species,[101] succinic acid was found to be the major product of fermentation.   Acetic acid was also excreted in considerable amounts but very little lactic acid; other 3- to 6-carbon acids were excreted in small amounts.

These variations may be due to differences in gas phase, for later experiments[364] showed that under anaerobic conditions more than twice as much succinate was produced as under aerobic conditions, a result undoubtedly due to the production of succinate from fumarate derived from CO_2-fixation (p. 79).

In *E. granulosus*, only the end-products of metabolism of the protoscoleces, fresh from the hydatid cyst, have been examined, so that essentially only the larval metabolism has been studied.   The end-products of metabolism are different under aerobic and anaerobic conditions, although the consumption of glycogen is not significantly different.   Under aerobic conditions the main product is lactic acid, with a lesser quantity of acetic acid, and small quantities of pyruvic and succinic acids, and some ethyl alcohol (Table 18).   Under anaerobic conditions no pyruvic acid is excreted, but more lactic acid is produced than under aerobiosis, and—as in *H. diminuta*—considerably more succinic acid (the equivalent of about 30% of the glycogen utilised) is released (Table 18).

Carbon dioxide is produced by all cestodes studied, but the fate of this gas has not been determined; some of it may be utilised for carbon dioxide fixation (p. 76).

Intermediary Metabolism
General Account

It is assumed that the reader is familiar with the general pattern of metabolic pathways in animal tissues, many of which also occur in plants, protozoa and bacteria.   Details of these pathways are given in most biochemistry texts.   Although the metabolic pathways of only a limited number of cestode species have been studied, the three metabolic pathways best known in most animal tissues occur also in cestodes, although in a somewhat modified form; these are (a) glycolysis (the Embden-Meyerhof pathway) (b) oxidative decarboxylation (the Krebs Cycle or citric acid cycle); (c) oxidative phosphorylation (the electron transport system; the cytochrome system). A further pathway, the hexose mono-phosphate shunt, has been described in some species.

The underlying function of these pathways is the production of energy-rich molecules of ATP (adenosine triphosphate) by the step-wise oxidation of glucose molecules to carbon dioxide. Hydrogen atoms involved in these reactions are transferred via various carrier molecules (e.g. NAD) to oxygen to form water.

The evidence for the existence of these pathways consists essentially of demonstration of the enzymatic steps and identification of the intermediate compounds in the pathway; inhibitors are often used to determine the former.

Glycolysis: the Embden-Meyerhof Pathway

In this pathway, the glucose molecule is broken down into two molecules of pyruvic acid, with the transfer of two pairs of hydrogen atoms to NAD. This process takes place not in one reaction but by a series of steps involving a succession of enzymes (Table 20), with the result that energy is released, in quantities small enough to be handled by the cell.

Nearly all the studies on enzymes in cestodes have been based on homogenates of tissue with the addition of co-factors such as ATP and NAD and catalytic ions such as Mg^{2+}. The enzymes of the Embden-Meyerhof pathway have been examined in detail only in *E. granulosus* and *H. diminuta*, with a few incidental observations on *Moniezia benedeni* and *Taenia crassiceps*.[285, 316] In *Hymenolepis*, the following enzymes have been demonstrated*: phosphorylase, phosphohexomutase, hexokinase, aldolase, phosphoglyceraldehyde dehydrogenase and lactic dehydrogenase.[297] A series of very detailed studies on the carbohydrate metabolism of the protoscolex stage of *Echinococcus* have been made by Agosin and his co-workers[1-9] and an excellent account of the biochemistry of this organism is available.[2] Essentially the *larval* metabolism was studied, but these results may give some general indication of the carbohydrate metabolism in the adult worm, although a switch-over of metabolic pathways in the adult worm may occur (p. 154). In homo-

* The nomenclature of enzymes has undergone some major changes in the last few years, as a result of recommendations by the Enzyme Commission[93], so that names previously in use will become obsolete. For convenience, the names of enzymes given by the original workers have been generally used in this text.

TABLE 20

Embden-Meyerhof pathway of anaerobic glycolysis*

1. Glycogen$+nH_3PO_4$ $\xrightarrow{\alpha\text{-glucan phosphorylase}}$ n glucose 1-phosphate

2. Glucose 1-phosphate+glucose 1, 6-diphosphate $\xrightleftharpoons{\text{Phosphoglucomutase}}$ glucose 1, 6-diphosphate+glucose 6-phosphate

Alternatively, starting with glucose, 1 and 2 are replaced by 3.

3. Glucose+ATP $\xrightarrow{\text{Hexokinase}}$ glucose 6-phosphate+ADP

4. Glucose 6-phosphate $\xrightleftharpoons{\text{Glucosephosphate isomerase}}$ fructose 6-phosphate

5. Fructose 6-phosphate+ATP $\xrightleftharpoons{\text{Phosphofructokinase}}$ fructose 1, 6-diphosphate +ADP

6. Fructose, 1, 6-diphosphate $\xrightleftharpoons{\text{Aldolase}}$ dihydroxyacetone phosphate+D-glyceraldehyde 3-phosphate

7. Dihydroxyacetone phosphate $\xrightleftharpoons{\text{Triosephosphate isomerase}}$ D-glyceraldehyde 3-phosphate

8. D-glyceraldehyde 3-phosphate+dehydrogenase+NAD
   $\xrightleftharpoons[\text{dehydrogenase}]{\text{Glyceraldehydephosphate}}$ 3-phospho-D-glyceric acid-enzyme complex
   $+NADH_2$

9. 3-phospho-D-glyceric acid-enzyme complex$+H_3PO_4$
   $\xrightleftharpoons[\text{dehydrogenase}]{\text{Glyceraldehydephosphate}}$ 1, 3-diphospho-D-glycerate+dehydrogenase

10. 1, 3-diphospho-D-glycerate+ADP $\xrightleftharpoons{\text{Phosphoglycerate kinase}}$ 3-phospho-D-glycerate+ATP

11. 3-phospho-D-glycerate+2, 3-diphospho-D-glycerate $\xrightleftharpoons{\text{Phosphoglyceromutase}}$ 2, 3-diphospho-D-glycerate+2-phospho-D-glycerate

12. 2-phospho-D-glycerate $\xrightleftharpoons{\text{Phosphopyruvate hydratase}}$ phosphoenol-pyruvate $+H_2O$

13. Phosphoenol-pyruvate+ADP $\xrightleftharpoons{\text{Pyruvate kinase}}$ pyruvate+ATP

If O_2 is absent, the $NADH_2$ from Reaction 8 is oxidized in muscle by Reaction 14 and the end-product is lactate:

14. Pyruvate $\xrightleftharpoons{\text{Lactate dehydrogenase}}$ L-lactate

Sum of reactions 3–14: glucose+2 ADP$+2H_3PO_4 = 2$ lactic acid+2 ATP $+2H_2O$

* Enzyme terminology as recommended by the Enzyme Commission.[93]

genates of *Echinococcus* protoscoleces, the following enzymes of the Embden-Meyerhof pathway have been identified: myokinase, phosphoglucomutase, phosphoglucose isomerase, phosphofructokinase, aldolase, glycerophosphate dehydrogenase and lactic dehydrogenase.[3]

Although these results have not enabled the identification of all the enzymes of the Embden-Meyerhof scheme, they do suggest that phosphorylative glycolysis occurs at least in the species studied and is probably the general pattern in cestodes.

Oxidative Decarboxylation: The Krebs (citric acid) Cycle

General account. Decarboxylation means the removal of the carboxyl group of an organic acid, often with the production of CO_2. In some organisms, such as yeast, 'straight' decarboxylation occurs which results in breaking up the carboxyl group to give CO_2:—

$$CH_3—CO—COOH \longrightarrow CH_3CHO + CO_2$$
pyruvic acid   acetaldehyde

$$CH_3 CHO + NADH_2 \longrightarrow CH_3—CH_2OH + NAD$$
acetaldehyde   ethyl alcohol

Since ethyl alcohol has been detected in the waste products of the metabolism of the protoscoleces of *E. granulosus*,[2] it is possible that this organism may partly utilise this simple form of decarboxylation. In the majority of organisms, however, oxidative decarboxylation occurs and use is made of oxygen (from water) according to the general equation:

$$R \cdot CO \cdot COOH + H_2O \longrightarrow R \cdot COOH + 2H + CO_2$$

the hydrogen atoms being removed by various hydrogen carrier molecules.

The Krebs cycle is made up of a sequence of reactions which include several such oxidative decarboxylation steps. This cycle has been shown to occur in many invertebrates, including other parasitic helminths such as nematodes [215a] and trematodes[422] although sometimes in a modified form. The significance of the cycle to an organism, however, is much greater than that indicated by the mere oxidation of pyruvic acid, for it is essentially the point at which the carbohydrate, fat and protein metabolisms can meet. Since α-ketoglutaric, oxaloacetic and pyruvic acids can readily be formed from the amino acids, glutamic acid, aspartic acid and alanine, respectively, the Krebs cycle is concerned also in the oxidation of some of the protein intermediates. In addition, many other amino acids can be broken down to substances which form intermediate products of the cycle, such as fumarate, succinate, oxaloacetate and α-ketoglutarate.   Acetyl-CoA, a key substance in the cycle, is also concerned in fat metabolism.

From these considerations it can be seen that most of the carbon atoms of the chemical constituents of tissue pass through the Krebs

TABLE 21

The Citric acid or Krebs cycle[*]

1. Acetyl-CoA+oxaloacetate $\xrightarrow{\text{Citrate synthase}}$ citrate+CoA

2. Citrate $\xrightarrow{\text{Aconitate hydratase}}$ cis-aconitate+H_2O

3. cis-aconitate+H_2O $\xrightarrow{\text{Aconitate hydratase}}$ L_S-isocitrate

4. L_S-isocitrate+NADP $\xrightarrow{\text{Isocitrate dehydrogenase}}$ oxalosuccinate+$NADPH_2$

5. $NADPH_2$+$\frac{1}{2}O_2$ $\xrightarrow{\text{NADPH}_2\ \text{cytochrome } c \text{ reductase}}$ $NADP$+H_2O
   and cytochrome oxidase

6. Oxalosuccinate $\xrightarrow{\text{Isocitrate dehydrogenase}}$ 2-oxoglutarate+CO_2

7. 2-oxoglutarate+oxidized lipoate $\xrightarrow{\text{Oxoglutarate dehydrogenase with thiamine}}$
   $\qquad\qquad\qquad\qquad\qquad\qquad\qquad\qquad\qquad\qquad$ pyrophosphate
   6-S-succinyl-hydrolipoate

8. 6-S-succinyl-hydrolipoate $\xrightarrow{\text{Lipoate acetyltransferase}}$ succinyl-CoA+
   dihydrolipoate

9. Succinyl-CoA+H_2O $\xrightarrow{\text{Succinyl-CoA hydrolase}}$ succinate+CoA

10. Succinate+$\frac{1}{2}O_2$ $\xrightarrow{\text{Succinate dehydrogenase and cytochrome oxidase}}$ fumarate
    +H_2O

11. Fumarate+H_2O $\xrightarrow{\text{Fumarate hydratase}}$ L-malate

12. L-malate+NAD $\xrightarrow{\text{Malate dehydrogenase}}$ oxaloacetate+$NADH_2$

Sum of reactions: Acetyl-CoA+$2O_2$=$2CO_2$+H_2O+CoA

[*] Enzyme terminology as recommended by the Enzyme Commission.[93]

cycle in some of its intermediates. The explanation for this is that the 4-carbon intermediates in particular are closely involved in other metabolic pathways, e.g. those concerned in the synthesis of the ribose material in the formation of nucleic acids.

Evidence for the Krebs cycle in cestodes. With the exception of *Echinococcus*, which is dealt with separately below, evidence for the existence of the enzymes of the Krebs cycle in cestodes is very incomplete. It is based for the most part on the histochemical demonstration of enzymes, such as succinic dehydrogenase, or the demonstration of oxidation of intermediates by homogenates. Such evidence must be further supported by a demonstration that the cycle is actually operative in the intact organism; for, as stressed elsewhere (p. 41), permeability barriers may serve to prevent such intermediates from reaching the enzyme sites *in vivo*.[8]

Histochemical methods have demonstrated succinic dehydrogenase in the larva and adult stages of a number of species (see Table 2). In addition, dehydrogenases capable of reducing isocitrate, glutamate, α-ketoglutarate, malate and lactate have been demonstrated histochemically in some of these species—*H. diminuta, H. nana, H. citelli, Hydatigera taeniaeformis*.[343] Histochemical results in general indicate that these enzymes are concentrated chiefly in the tegument, thus confirming the metabolic importance of this region.

Experiments with homogenates of cestodes have also demonstrated the oxidation of succinic acid in *Taenia pisiformis*;[284, 316] *Moniezia benedeni*;[134] *H. diminuta*[299] and *H. nana*.[121] The oxidation of malic and glutamic acids and the conversion of fumaric acid to malic acid has also been reported for homogenates of *H. diminuta*.[300]

Although this evidence for these species is suggestive, in no instance has the function of the enzymes concerned been demonstrated in the *intact* organism. Studies on *Echinococcus*, however, provide strong evidence of the functioning of a Krebs cycle in this species. Thus, it was shown (Table 22) that a number of Krebs cycle intermediates were oxidised both in intact protoscoleces and whole homogenates. Cell free preparations were found to contain a condensing enzyme, a NADP- and a NAD-dependent isocitric dehydrogenase, succinic, malic and α-ketoglutaric dehydrogenases, as well as fumarase, aconitase, pyruvic oxidase and α-carboxylase. It is interesting to note that in these results (Table 22) the three intermediates which failed to be oxidised by the intact protoscoleces—pyruvate, α-ketoglutarate and lactate—were oxidised by homogenates. This may indicate that only an incomplete cycle operates; alternatively it may support the point made above, viz. that permeability barriers may have prevented the substrate reaching the enzyme sites in the intact animal.

It is curious to note, however, that, in contrast, both succinate and glycollate were oxidised as rapidly in intact protoscoleces as in the homogenates.

TABLE 22

Oxidation of Krebs cycle intermediates by Echinococcus granulosus *intact protoscoleces and* 0·25 M *sucrose homogenates*
(Data from Agosin & Repetto[8])

Substrate	Intact protoscoleces : oxygen uptake μl/100 mg. dry wt./hour	Whole homogenates: oxygen uptake μl/mg. N/hour
Pyruvate	0·0	31
Citrate	1·0	0·0
Fumarate	21·0	2·0
Malate	39·0	55·0
Isocitrate	62·0	344
α-ketoglutarate	0·0	50
Oxaloacetate	32·0	0·0
Acetate	13·0	8
Succinate	200·0	94
Glutamate	39·0	58
Glyoxylate	27·0	113
Glycollate	193·0	2·0
Lactate	0·0	41·0

In *Echinococcus* then, and probably in the species listed above, a Krebs cycle operates in whole or in part. It does not necessarily follow that this pattern of metabolism is followed in all cestodes; for it has been shown in parasitic nematodes that, although the Krebs cycle operates in many species, it does not do so in all.[215a]

CO_2-*Fixation in Cestodes*

General account. Somewhat related to the Krebs cycle is the problem of CO_2-fixation by cestodes. It has already been pointed out that CO_2 has a remarkable effect in stimulating glycogenesis and glucose utilisation in *H. diminuta* (Table 15); moreover, the production of succinic acid was increased seven-fold when CO_2 was present.[101] Formation of succinic acid in metabolism commonly entails CO_2-fixation, and since this substance is produced by species such as *H. diminuta* and *E. granulosus* it was conjectured that CO_2-fixation occurs in both these organisms. Experimental work especially with $^{14}CO_2$, confirms this view.[8, 9, 51, 101]

As carbon dioxide fixation is not a common phenomenon in animal tissues, it is of especial interest to examine the biochemistry of the process in some detail. The discovery of CO_2-fixation in animal tissues arose from studies carried out on the fate of pyruvic acid in pigeon liver—

a tissue known to be capable of synthesising a 5-carbon chain (e.g. α-ketoglutaric acid, $COOH.CO.CH_2 CH_2 COOH$) from added pyruvic acid, a 3-carbon acid. This curious ability of pigeon liver to form ketoglutarate from pyruvate without the addition of a dicarboxylic acid led to the idea that this tissue is capable of synthesising oxaloacetic acid (an important intermediate product in the Krebs cycle) from pyruvate and CO_2. Experiments on this and other tissues, especially with tracer techniques, has fully confirmed this hypothesis. More extensive work has shown that the following five primary fixation reactions can occur in animal tissues:

(a) CO_2+pyruvic acid——→oxaloacetic acid
(b) CO_2+pyruvic acid——→malic acid
(c) CO_2+ketoglutaric acid——→oxalosuccinic acid
(d) ornithine+CO_2+NH_3——→citrulline
(e) CO_2+glycine+formic acid+NH_3——→hypoxanthine.

There is evidence that in some species of nematodes[204] fumarate, an intermediary in the sequence of reactions, pyruvate+CO_2——→ succinate, serves as a hydrogen acceptor (or as an oxidiser) for the reoxidation of NADH a substance involved in glycolysis and glycogenesis.

$$
\begin{array}{ccccc}
& COOH & COOH & COOH & COOH \\
CH_3 & | & | & | & | \\
| & CH_2 & CH_2 & CH & CH_2 \\
+CO_2 & | & | & | & | \\
CO \xrightarrow{} & | \underset{\longrightarrow}{+2H} & | \underset{\longrightarrow}{-H_2O} & | \underset{\longrightarrow}{+2H} & | \\
| & CO & CHOH & CH & CH_2 \\
COOH & | & | & | & | \\
& COOH & COOH & COOH & COOH \\
\text{pyruvic} & \text{oxaloacetic} & \text{malic} & \text{fumaric} & \text{succinic} \\
\text{acid} & \text{acid} & \text{acid} & \text{acid} & \text{acid}
\end{array}
$$

Thus, a CO_2 lack could lead to a deficiency in fumarate, and this would adversely affect the reoxidation of NADH (Fig. 28) and so inhibit glycogenesis.[101] This would account for the value of CO_2 in *in vitro* culture (Chapter 10).

CO_2-Fixation in Echinococcus granulosus

Succinic acid is one of the major metabolic end-products in *Echinococcus* (Table 18), a fact which suggests that CO_2-fixation is taking place. It was also found that this organism could utilise

[14]C-labelled CO_2 for the synthesis of Krebs cycle intermediates: proteins, lipids and phospholipids, nucleic acids and polysaccharides[8] (Fig. 24). The actual distribution in the various cellular fractions is given in Table 23.

TABLE 23

Distribution in cellular fractions of radiocarbon from [14]CO_2
utilised by intact E. granulosus *protoscoleces*
(Data from Agosin & Repetto[8])

Fraction	Radioactivity (c.p.m./100 mg. dry weight)	
	12 hr.	24 hr.
Acid soluble (cold TCA)	218,000	278,000
Ethanol soluble	3,920	5,700
Ether soluble	1,330	1,490
Alkali soluble	18,960	8,550
Hot acid soluble	1,090	1,800
Protein	1,800	4,420
Total	245,100	299,960

After twenty-four hours' incubation of intact protoscoleces, some 93% of the ^{14}C appeared in the acid-soluble fraction; 1·5% in the

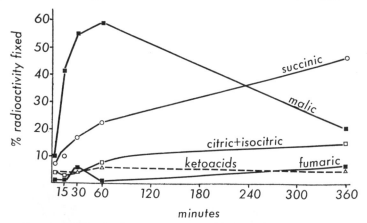

FIG. 24. [14]CO_2-fixation into organic acids by *Echinococcus granulosus* protoscoleces. (After Agosin & Repetto, 1965.)

protein fraction and about 8% in the hot acid-soluble fraction (presumably phospholipids and peptides). Of the acid-soluble fraction, 70% of the ^{14}C was found in succinic acid, 1% in lactic acid and 1% in volatile fatty acids. CO_2 was also utilised for polysaccharide synthesis, the polysaccharide isolated from protoscoleces being found to contain 7% of the original $^{14}CO_2$ utilised. When the pathways followed after CO_2-fixation were further examined[9] it was found that in *homogenates* of protoscoleces four mechanisms for CO_2-fixation could be demonstrated:

(a) Phosphoenol Pyruvic Acid $+ CO_2 + \dfrac{GDP}{(IDP)} \xrightleftharpoons{\text{PEP-carboxykinase}} OAA + \dfrac{GTP*}{(ITP)}$

(b) $PEP + CO_2 \xrightarrow{\text{PEP-carboxylase}} OAA + Pi$

(c) Pyruvate $+ CO_2 + \dfrac{CTP}{(ATP)} \xrightleftharpoons{\text{pyruvate carboxylase}} OAA + \dfrac{CDP}{(ATP)} + Pi$

(d) Pyruvate $+ CO_2 + NADPH + H^+ \xrightleftharpoons{\text{'malic enzyme'}} malate + NADP$

Abbreviations:

CTP,	cytosine triphosphate;	GDP,	guanosine diphosphate;
*GTP,	guanosine triphosphate;	IDP,	inosine diphosphate;
ITP,	inosine triphosphate;	OAA,	oxaloacetic acid;
PEP,	phospho(enol) pyruvic acid;	Pi,	inorganic phosphorus

* An alternative high energy carrier which replaces ATP in protein synthesis.

Of these four enzyme systems, however, only PEP-carboxykinase and 'malic enzyme' show a sufficiently high activity to account for the production of succinate *in vitro*. Thus, in three hours 0·0963 μ mole oxaloacetic acid/mg protein is formed under conditions appropriate for PEP-carboxykinase activity, in the presence of inosine diphosphate;[9] this figure corresponds to 8·91 μ moles succinate/g fresh weight/per 3 hr. This activity could more than account for the total production of succinate by protoscoleces—approximately 7·0 μ moles/g fresh weight/3 hr. under anaerobic conditions. On the other hand, the activity of the 'malic enzyme' has been shown to be much higher[8] and could produce 72 μ moles succinate/g fresh weight/ 3 hr.—which strongly suggests that the 'malic enzyme' is the primary enzyme system concerned in succinate production. It should be pointed out, however, that some succinate is also produced by another pathway—further discussed below.

CO_2-Fixation in Hymenolepis diminuta

Isotope studies have shown that CO_2-fixation pathways comparable to those occurring in *E. granulosus*, occur also in *H. diminuta*.[290, 364] The most active CO_2-fixing enzyme is again PEP-carboxylase which appears to be localised mainly in the soluble fraction, with some activity in the particulate fraction. Some further CO_2-fixation takes place via the ' malic enzyme ' which activity is associated with the particulate fraction. The amount of $^{14}CO_2$ fixed is sufficient to account for the amount of succinic acid formed under anaerobic conditions.[364] As in *Echinococcus*, some fixed CO_2 was also incorporated into polysaccharide,[307] although the precise link between CO_2-fixation and glycogenesis is not clear.

Although the main incorporation of ^{14}C in these experiments was into succinate and/or fumarate, as in *Echinococcus*, incorporation into lactate, pyruvate, malate and oxaloacetate also occurred. Additional confirmation of the labelling of the keto acids was obtained by determining the incorporation into free amino acids. Because of transaminase activity (p. 92) in *Hymenolepis*, incorporation into either alanine, aspartate or glutamate reflects incorporation into the corresponding keto acid. The majority of ^{14}C was incorporated into alanine.[290]

The Pentose Phosphate Pathway

Although the Embden-Meyerhof pathway of glycolysis undoubtedly represents the main route of the conversion of carbohydrates to pyruvic acid in animal tissues, it is by no means the only metabolic pathway by which carbohydrate can be utilised. Experimentally, the occurrence of alternative pathways is indicated if it is found that inhibitors such as arsenite, fluoride or iodoacetate—which block component reactions in the Embden-Meyerhof pathway—fail to block glucose utilisation completely. One such alternative pathway which occurs in plants, some animal tissues and some microorganisms, involves the oxidation of glucose-6-phosphate to 6-phosphogluconic acid, which is converted to pentose phosphates (Fig. 25). This route is known by a number of names: the ' pentose phosphate pathway ', the ' hexose monophosphate oxidation shunt' or the 'Warburg-Dickens pathway.' The term *pentose phosphate pathway* is used here. Pathways other than the glycolytic or pentose pathways are known in other biological systems but have not been investigated in cestodes. Briefly, the first step in the pentose phosphate pathway involves oxidation of glucose-6-phosphate to the corresponding 6-phosphogluconic acid. The electron acceptor is NADP, not NAD. The remainder of the pathway is shown in Fig. 25. The system basically involves the total oxidation of a glucose molecule to CO_2.

During each oxidative decarboxylation, carbon 1 of the hexose is converted to CO_2; when the remaining carbons of the glucose molecules pass through the cycle, each one is successively transformed to carbon 1 of fructose-6-phosphate and then removed by oxidative decarboxylation.

The occurrence of the pentose phosphate pathway is well known in nematodes,[215a] and it has been demonstrated that it occurs, in whole or in part, in several species of cestodes. Thus, in *Anoplocephala perfoliata, Moniezia benedeni, T. saginata, T. pisiformis* and *Dipylidium caninum*, the occurrence of two enzymes of the pentose phosphate cycle, glucose-6-phosphate dehydrogenase and gluconate-6-phosphate dehydrogenase, has been demonstrated; moreover, in all cases the enzymes

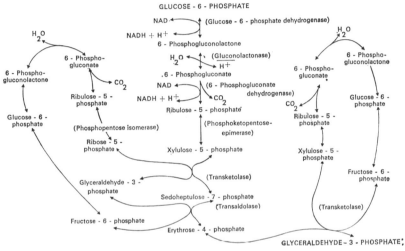

FIG. 25. Schematic representation of the pentose phosphate pathway. (After Patton, 1963, from Gilmour.)

were NADP-dependent.[220]   The pathway appears to be absent in *H. diminuta*.[364]   Evidence for the existence of a complete pentose phosphate cycle in larval *E. granulosus* has been provided by Agosin and his co-workers.[5, 7]

Analysis of extra-corporeal fluid of *E. granulosus* during endogenous polysaccharide utilisation showed the presence of glucose, fructose, ribose, ribulose, sedoheptulose and glyceraldehyde. Since ribose, ribulose and sedoheptulose are intermediates of the pentose phosphate pathway, it was speculated that this pathway operated, to some extent, in this species. More detailed studies[5] confirmed the existence of many of the enzymes of the pentose phosphate pathway in cell-free extracts, *viz* glucose-6-phosphate and 6-phosphogluconic dehydrogenases, transketolase, transaldolase, phosphopentose isomerase, ribokinase, 3-phosphoglyceraldehyde dehydrogenase, triosephosphate isomerase and (possibly) phosphoketopentose epimerase.

The question can now be asked, how important is the pentose phosphate sequence in *Echinococcus*? By the use of labelled carbon it has been shown that about 60% of glucose utilised by this species is metabolised by the Embden-Meyerhof pathway, some 20% by the pentose phosphate pathway and the remaining 20% by non-triose pathways, at present unknown. It would be most interesting to determine the nature of these unknown alternative pathways.

Glycerol Absorption and Utilisation

The apparent importance of the carbohydrate metabolism has probably led to other possible energy substrates being overlooked. For example, it has been shown that the polyhydric alcohol, glycerol, can be absorbed by both larval and adult *H. taeniaeformis*.[39] Since in many animal tissues this substance can be degraded by means of the glycolytic pathway, this finding is of interest. Mutual inhibition between glycerol and glucose uptake did not occur.

Electron Transport

The Embden-Meyerhof pathway and the Krebs cycle result essentially in oxidation of all the carbon atoms of the carbohydrate molecule to CO_2, and for each glucose molecule we are left with a total of twelve pairs of hydrogen atoms (two from the Embden-Meyerhof cycle and ten from the Krebs cycle), ten of which are in the care of NAD or NADP. In the systems which have been most thoroughly studied, yeast and vertebrate muscle and liver, the hydrogen atoms are transferred to flavoproteins (which have as their prosthetic group flavin adenine dinucleotide (FAD)), lose electrons and become hydrogen ions. The electrons are passed to a complex ' cytochrome system ', comprising at least five cytochromes b, c_1, c, a, and a_3 (cytochrome oxidase) and finally to molecular O_2 to form water (Fig. 26). This respiratory chain is known as the *electron transport system*, and its enzymes appear to be located in the inner membranes of the mitochondria.

Although the basic principles of the mammalian electron transport system are well established, there is considerable disagreement on many important details.[17] It is not surprising, therefore, to find that the electron transport system in cestodes—which is much more difficult to investigate—is very poorly known.

The cytochrome system described above is essentially an *aerobic* system, and can operate satisfactorily only at an oxygen tension not less than 5 mm. Hg.[84] Since the majority of cestode strobila occur in the paramucosa (p. 2) where the oxygen tension approaches zero,

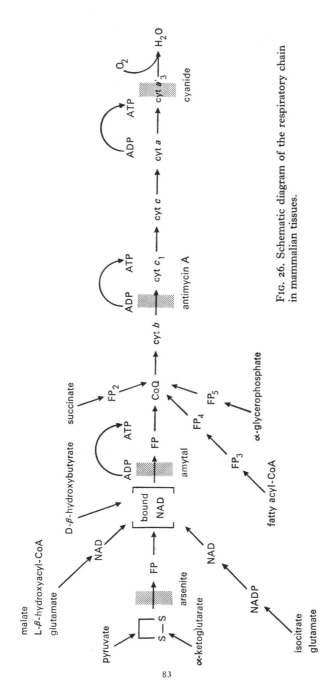

83

Fig. 26. Schematic diagram of the respiratory chain in mammalian tissues.

it is doubtful whether such an electron transport system can operate at all in cestodes. Evidence from other helminth parasites, especially nematodes such as *Ascaris*, suggests that the terminal respiration sequence in such groups may be considerably modified.[204, 215a]

Detection of the components of an electron transport system, involving cytochrome systems, is based on (*a*) identification of the various cytochromes by absorption and difference spectroscopy, and (*b*) the use of 'specific' inhibitors for the various stages of transference— especially involving succinic dehydrogenase and cytochrome oxidase. Such results, by themselves, must be interpreted with caution, for it is difficult to demonstrate unequivocally the specificity of such inhibitors. Thus, it is generally accepted that the reversal of CO-inhibition by light is the most specific test for cytochrome oxidase, and yet there are many oxidases which show this behaviour, and have an absorption at 600 mμ, yet do not oxidise cytochrome.[17]

Cyanide has been found to inhibit aerobic respiration in *D. latum*,[108] *E. granulosus*,[6] *H. diminuta*,[316] *Triaenophorus lucii*,[108] *Moniezia benedeni*,[134] and *Hydatigera taeniaeformis*;[316] which suggests that aerobic respiration involves enzyme systems containing heavy metals, possibly a cytochrome system. On the other hand, respiration in *D. latum* and *T. lucii* is not inhibited by carbon monoxide[108] which blocks cytochrome oxidase; this suggests that these species do not contain cytochrome oxidase or that they possss an alternative oxidase. However, spectra characteristic of cytochromes have been demonstrated with tissues of *D. latum*, *T. lucii*[108] and *M. benedeni*.[134] Again, in *H. diminuta* direct or indirect evidence has indicated the presence of a cytochrome oxidase[299] and a cytochrome *c* reductase which utilises NADH, NADPH or succinate as hydrogen donors.[300, 316] A catalase and a peroxidase have also been identified in larval and adult *Taenia pisiformis* and in *M. expansa*,[60, 284]

None of the above evidence is sufficiently unequivocal to indicate that a cytochrome system of the usual type operates in cestodes. Detailed studies on particulate fractions, rich in mitochondria, of *Moniezia expansa* and *Taenia hydatigena* with low temperature (77°K) spectroscopy has indicated the existence of an unusual form of electron transport pathway involving cytochromes of the *b* group, which is probably closely related to that present in *Ascaris*.[58, 61, 62, 215a] The main cytochrome component in *Moniezia* was found to be of the '*b*' type with a wavelength of 557 mμ (Fig. 27); small amounts of cytochrome *a* were also present, and cytochrome *c* was not at first detected. Later, very low levels of c_1 and *c* cytochromes were identified. Cyanide or carbon monoxide did not inhibit succinate oxidation. Manometric experiments with dyes and inhibitors led to the conclusions (*a*) that cytochrome c and cytochrome oxidase are either absent in this species or present in small amounts and are not concerned with the anaerobic oxidation of succinate and NADH; (b) that at least one cytochrome of the group b is present, but is probably not involved in *aerobic* respiration, and (c) that oxidation of NADH proceeds by a separate pathway.

The appearance of hydrogen peroxide in experiments with particulate fractions under aerobic conditions led to the hypothesis that under

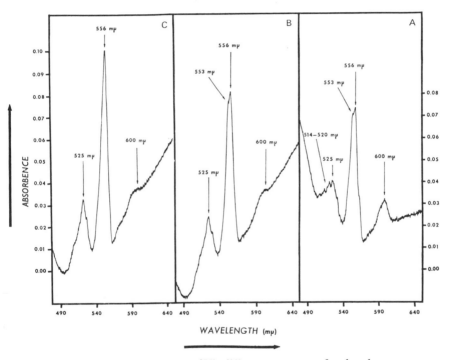

Fig. 27. Low-temperature (77°K) difference spectra of reduced cytochromes and flavoproteins in a particulate fraction of *Moniezia expansa*. A. Reduction with succinate only. B. Reduction with succinate plus dithionite. C. Effect of addition of ferricyanide after treatment as in B. (After Cheah & Bryant, 1966.)

these conditions the oxidation of NADH and succinate in *M. expansa* is mediated by flavoproteins with the accumulation of hydrogen peroxide, the cytochrome b (557) apparently not playing any role in this system. It seems unlikely that, in the natural environment, the oxygen tension would be sufficiently high for this system to operate, and it must therefore, be regarded as largely an artificial system.[62]

On the other hand, the occurrence of a peroxidase in *Monieza* may indicate that some peroxide (which is biologically toxic) is formed *in vivo* and is removed by this enzyme.[59]

The metabolic pathway believed to be followed by *Moniezia* under *anaerobic* conditions, is shown in Fig. 28. This is essentially a process whereby the NADH formed during glycolysis can be reoxidised by an electron transport system which involves cytochrome b (557) and flavoprotein carriers, with fumarate, which is reduced to succinate, as the terminal acceptor. Thus this electron transport system provides

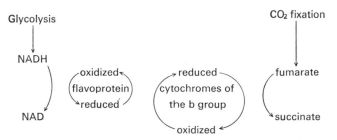

Fig. 28. Possible form of electron transport system in *Moniezia expansa*. (see p. 84)

a mechanism for oxidising NADH under anaerobic conditions. It also accounts for the excretion of succinate by *Moniezia* under anaerobic conditions. Much of the fumarate utilised in this system may come from CO_2-fixation (see p. 76). A comparable system may operate in both larval and adult *E. granulosus*.[47]

More recent work has shown that electron transport in *M. expansa* is more complex than appears from the above studies.

6: The Adult: Protein and Lipid Metabolism

Protein Composition

Protein Content

The protein content of animal tissue is generally based on the total nitrogen content, multiplying the latter by a factor of 6·25. This factor is based on analysis of mammalian tissue, and takes into account the average nitrogen content of the main acids making up tissue protein. Although this figure holds for some species of cestodes, it does not hold for all of them, because of a relatively high proportion of non-protein nitrogen. Thus, for larval and adult *Hydatigera taeniaeformis* it has been shown that the observed and ' calculated ' (i.e. the total of its constituents) figures for dry weight coincide closely.[38] Since these values are related to the calculated total protein content, it can be argued that, at least for this species, the conversion factor of 6·25 cannot be grossly inaccurate. In contrast, in some species a substantial proportion of the nitrogen in the total nitrogen figure is in the non-protein fraction. Thus, in *Moniezia expansa, Thysanosoma actinioides* and *Cittotaenia perplexa* the non-protein nitrogen varied between 9 and 16% of the total nitrogen and the total protein content varied between 20 and 29% of the dry weight respectively (Table 9); these latter values are lower than those previously reported in cestodes. *T. saginata* has also been shown to contain significant quantities of non-protein nitrogen.[235] Earlier figures for ' protein ' in cestodes (Table 9), should therefore, be accepted with caution, until the level of non-protein nitrogen is known.

Fractionation of tissue proteins of cestodes has been carried out in only a few species—*Echinococcus granulosus*;[75, 289] *Moniezia expansa*;[190] *Hymenolepis diminuta*;[192, 193] *T. saginata*;[235] some of these proteins are unusual in that they have been found to be conjugated with other tissue substances such as glycogen, cerebrosides, or bile acids. The significance of such complexes in cestode tissue has yet to be determined.

The structural proteins reported in cestodes are keratin, which makes up the hooks and embryophores in taeniid cestodes, and sclerotin (tanned protein), which forms the egg capsules in Pseudophyllidea and possibly other groups (p. 112).   Keratin is a protein in which the molecules are cross-linked with the sulphur-containing amino acid cystine (Fig. 40).   The hooks and the embryophore blocks (p. 115) of a number of cyclophyllid species have been shown to give histochemical reactions and to have chemical and physical properties consistent with those of a keratin-type protein.[110, 249]   The amino acid composition (Table 24) of the embryophore is similar to that of vertebrate keratin.   The high sulphur content, which is related to a high cystine content, is particularly significant.   In *Echinococcus*, the hooks contained 15·6% N and 5·6% S;[110] in the embryophores of *Taenia* spp., the corresponding analyses were 12·1–14·2% N and 2·0–3·0% S.[249]   These figures may be compared with the following analyses of sheep wool: 16·2–16·9% N; 3·0–4·0% S.[249]   Infrared analyses carried out on embryophores gave spectra with absorption peaks almost identical with those of vertebrate keratins, for which the characteristic peaks occur at 3300 cm^{-1}, 1650 cm^{-1}, and 1540^{-1}.

TABLE 24

Amino acids in the proteins of the blocks of embryophores of taeniid cestodes, compared with those of vertebrate keratin
(Data from Morseth[249])

Amino acid	T. hydatigena	T. ovis	T. pisiformis	Keratin (ox horn)
Alanine	+	+	+	+
Arginine	+	+	+	+
Aspartic acid	+	+	+	+
Cysteic acid	?	?	?	?
Cystine*	+	+	+	+
Glutamic acid	+	+	+	+
Glycine	+	+	+	+
Histidine*	+	+	+	+
Isoleucine	(Not resolved	+	(Not resolved	(Not resolved
Leucine	into 2 separate spots)	+	into 2 separate spots)	into 2 separate spots)
Lysine	+	+	+	+
Methionine*	+	+	+	+
Phenylalanine*	+	+	+	+
Proline*	+	+	+	+
Serine	+	+	+	+
Threonine	+	+	+	+
Tryptophan*	+	+	−	−
Tyrosine*	+	+	+	+
Valine	+	+	+	+

* Identified by means of specific colour reagents.

Amino Acid Analysis

The amino acids occurring in the tissues of a number of adult and larval cestodes have been examined, and data are available for *H. diminuta*;[10, 127, 129] *M. expansa, Thysanosoma actinioides, Cittotaenia perplexa*;[52] *Anoplocephala magna*;[207] *E. granulosus*;[208] *T. saginata*;[235] *T. crassiceps*.[451] Results of analysis of the same species by different workers have not always been in agreement, probably because of variations of technique. In adults and cysticercoids of *H. diminuta*, it has been shown[129] that a close parallel exists between deficiency, or abundance, of amino acids in adults or cysticercoids and in intestinal tissue of the definitive rat host, or the tissues of the intermediate insect host (*Tribolium*), respectively. For example, aspartic acid, proline and hydroxyproline were abundant in adult worms and rats, but present only in decreased amounts in cysticercoids and beetles; on the other hand, the relative distribution of serine was reversed.

In addition to the better known amino acids, several uncommon ones have been reported in cestodes, namely β-alanine, [52, 208] β-amino-isobutyric acid and γ-aminobutyric acid.[52] There is some evidence that the first two of these are end-products of uracil and thymine degradation in this worm.[51]

Protein Metabolism

General Comments

Since protein forms a substantial part of the normal diet of a vertebrate, the intestine provides, for cestodes, an environment rich in proteins and related breakdown products, polypeptides, dipeptides and amino acids. As stressed earlier (Chapter 3), our concept of the nature of the intestinal environment—especially with regard to the extent to which the amino acid composition of the intestine fluctuates—has undergone a profound change within recent years.

Although it has been assumed by most workers on cestode physiology that only molecules of the size approaching those of amino acids can be absorbed by cestodes (through the tegument), it is now known that large molecules—such as dipeptides or even whole protein molecules—may be ingested. For this to occur, the cestode tegument must be capable of pinocytosis and we have no unequivocal experimental evidence (as yet!) that this is the case (p. 13) although ultrastructure studies are suggestive (Frontispiece). It is known that the normal intestinal mucosal cell, to which the cestode tegument shows considerable resemblance (Fig. 3), is probably capable of taking in dipeptides and that in the intestine of some newly born vertebrates whole protein molecules, such as immunoglobulins (p. 200), can be transported without previous breakdown.

Since some cestodes, e.g. *Echinococcus* (pp. 182-4), appear to be able to absorb material from the mucosal surface, it may be that a special form of digestion, namely ' membrane digestion[457] ' can occur. In this process the digestive enzyme is present on or in the membrane (i.e. it is membrane-bound) where the actual breakdown occurs. Again, it may be that proteins are actively digested at the host/parasite interface. In this situation, it is envisaged (Fig. 76) that the cestode cuticle releases proteolytic enzymes at its surface, these digest the proteins with which it is in contact, and the amino acids resulting are then absorbed by the tegument. The ' globular ' substructure (Fig. 4) of the plasma membranes covering the microtriches is further suggestive evidence that such a secretory process is taking place. Pinocytosis of whole protein may also possibly be involved (p. 13). Proteolytic enzymes have also been reported from *D. latum, E. granulosus, Taenia* spp.,[316] although whether these are extracellular or intracellular enzymes is not known.

Amino Acid Absorption

Studies with labelled compounds have shown that the uptake of amino acids by cestodes takes place by active transport.* Early work with *H. diminuta*[88-90] and *Raillietina cesticillus*[90] suggested that this was so, but the first unequivocal evidence appeared when it was shown[317-8] that *Calliobothrium verticillatum* accumulated L-valine against a concentration gradient. This process was a rapid one, the concentration difference of free L-valine, inside to outside, reaching ratios varying from 2·6: 1 to 4·3: 1 after forty minutes' incubation. Moreover, the Lineweaver-Burk reciprocal plot (1/V against 1/S, Fig. 29), was linear (i.e. the rate of uptake was non-linear with respect to medium concentration.)

Further evidence that active transport is involved in amino acid uptake by *Calliobothrium* is presented by the fact that the uptake of labelled L-valine or L-leucine was inhibited by a number of amino acids.[317] This result is accounted for by assuming that certain amino acids compete for the same ' carrier ' in the membrane transport system.

These early results, in general, have been confirmed in a number of other species. In *H. diminuta*, extensive studies with single and complex mixtures of amino acids[198, 314] have shown that at least four qualitatively different amino acid absorption loci occur in this worm. Some amino acids inhibit the uptake of others, whereas some have no

* As an understanding of active transport is of especial importance in cestode physiology, a brief theoretical account of this process is given in an appendix to this chapter

effect. This is interpreted as being due to competition for loci and the subsequent ' carrier ' mechanism in some cases and not in others. For example, in this species, lysine and arginine do not compete for the same locus. The degree of competition may be dependent on the absolute concentration of amino acids as well as their molar ratios.[198] Various substances, which have a molecular configuration sufficiently close to that of an amino acid, can act as an inhibitor for its uptake,

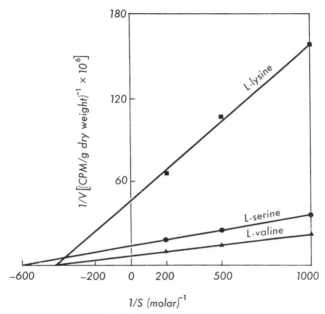

Fig. 29. Absorption of three ^{14}C-labelled amino acids by *Calliobothrium verticillatum* as a function of their external concentration. Lineweaver-Burk reciprocal plot of velocity (V) against amino acid concentration (S) expressed as counts per minute (CPM) per gram dry weight of worm. (After Read, Simmons, Campbell & Rothman, 1960.) (see p. 90.)

presumably by competing for the same locus. Comparable studies have been carried out on *H. citelli* in which it was found that each of fifteen different amino acids acted as a competitive inhibitor of methionine absorption. It was [378] further shown that the locus involved in methionine permeation requires that the amino group be in the alpha position to the carboxyl group.

These findings in respect to amino acid uptake by cestodes and competition for transport sites have implications with respect to the ecology of cestodes.[314, 378]   It has been emphasised that the molar ratios (but not the concentrations) of amino acids in the gut are relatively constant[266, 267]. In a particular host, a cestode is exposed to a relatively constant amino acid ratio to which its physiology would, undoubtedly, become adapted. In the ' wrong ' host, the required molar ratios of amino acids may not occur, and so growth of the worm may be inhibited; this ratio may thus be a factor in determining host specificity.

In the intestine, the molar ratios of amino acids in the lumen appear to be maintained partly by movement of amino acids from the mucosa into the lumen[403] but probably the pancreatic and duodenal secretions also contribute to the amino acid pool. In cestodes, a two-way traffic in amino acids undoubtedly occurs and a loss of amino acids may take place in certain environments. Thus, it has been shown that methionine is lost at a greater rate from *H. diminuta* in saline+amino acids than in saline alone—a phenomenon probably due to the stimulation of an outward flow of methionine by the uptake of other amino acids.[167]

Intermediary Metabolism

Amino acid requirements. As indicated above, cestodes readily absorb amino acids from the external environment under suitable physiological conditions. Certain amino acids can, however, be synthesised metabolically from other amino acids, and such amino acids are termed ' non-essential ' in contrast to those ' essential ' amino acids which the organism cannot synthesise and which must be present in the diet for normal growth.

Nothing appears to be known regarding the precise amino acid requirements in cestodes, or whether certain amino acids are 'essential ' or not. Studies of this nature are now technically possible, since many species can be cultured to maturity *in vitro* (Chapter 10). Little seems to be known, too, regarding the incorporation of absorbed amino acids into cestode proteins. Tracer studies have shown that tritiated proline is taken up first by the tegumental cells in the sub-cuticle and later incorporated into the distal cytoplasm of the tegument.[229]

Transamination. Although *H. diminuta* is capable of incorporating NH_4^+ ions into amino acids (Table 25) the main mechanism of amino acid synthesis appears to be transamination. In this process, the α-amino nitrogen of one amino acid is transferred, by means of specific enzymes, directly to a keto acid which forms a substrate for the formation of the new acid. The most studied systems are:

(i) α-ketoglutaric acid $\xrightarrow{\text{transaminase}}$ glutamic acid,

(ii) pyruvic acid $\xrightarrow{\text{transaminase}}$ alanine.

In both these systems, a number of amino acids can serve as amino group donors; other, less active, donors are purines and pyrimidines. Other ketoacids, such as oxaloacetic, can also act as transamination substrates, and this substance has been found to be so utilised in *H. diminuta*.[10] The α-ketoglutaric acid/glutamic acid system has

TABLE 25

Amino acid synthesis in Hymenolepis diminuta *from ammonia ; measurement in terms of amino nitrogen, in mg. produced by* 1 *gram worm* (*d.w.*)/*hr.*
(Data from Daugherty[86])

Incubation media	Amino N.
Krebs Ringer Phosphate	0·13
+(NH$_4$)$_2$ CO$_3$	1·4
+ α−ketoglutarate	4·8
+pyruvate	6·3
+oxaloacetate	7·4
+glucose	2·8
+succinate	2·4
+glucose+malonate	2·6

been shown to occur in three species of *Hymenolepis*[477] (Table 26) in *R. cestillus*[106] and in *Anoplocephala magna*.[207] The pyruvic acid/ alanine system has also been demonstrated in *Hymenolepis* spp., and in *R. cesticillus* (Table 26).[106, 477] Some seventeen amino acids failed to act as amino donors in either of these systems in *Hymenolepis*; which indicates that, compared with vertebrates, these species have an extremely limited capacity for performing transaminations. This result could be accounted for[477] by the fact that cestodes live in an environment rich in amino acids, in which case synthesis may play only a minor role in satisfying essential amino acid requirements.

Uptake of purines and pyrimidines. Since animal and plant material form a substantial part of the diet of vertebrates, it can be expected that break-down products of cell nuclei will be generally available to cestodes. For this reason, experiments on the uptake of purines and pyrimidines are of special interest. In extensive experiments on vertebrate tissues, such as kidney tubules or blood cells, it has been shown that (*a*) purines and pyrimidines can enter cells either by active transport sites or by facilitated diffusion (= mediated transport) in most organisms, (*b*) the transport sites in most organisms have a high affinity for hypoxanthine, which thus acts as a powerful inhibitor; (*c*) there are reciprocal inhibitions between purines and pyrimidines.[236]

In *H. diminuta* it has been found that the ' saturation kinetics ' (p. 103), such as apply to amino acid uptake in vertebrate tissues, do not apply. In the case of hypoxanthine, adenine and uracil, plots of velocity of uptake against substrate concentration (Figs. 30–32), show that the systems involved did not become saturated at the concentrations used.[236] Uptake of thymine and cytosine was shown to be a linear function of the concentration; which suggests that uptake of these substances took place by diffusion.[236] As is clear from Fig. 31, the

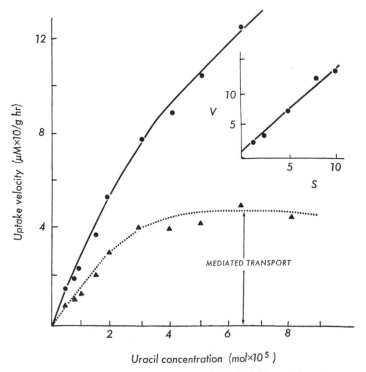

FIG. 30. Uptake of uracil by *Hymenolepis diminuta*. The upper curve represents observed values at high concentrations used to determine diffusion rate (slope=14). The lower curve represents total uptake minus the diffusion component, i.e. the area below the lower curve is considered as mediated transport. Inset: $V=$ uptake velocity in $\mu M/g$ hr; $S=$ uracil concentration in molarity 10^4. (After MacInnis, *et al.*, 1965.)

rate of uptake of adenine is linear in the range of concentrations used; this points to entry by diffusion. However, with this substance, and with uracil (Fig. 33), part of the uptake can be inhibited; from which it is concluded that part of the entry takes place by mediated transport.

It is interesting to note that the purine-pyrimidine transport locus in this organism is distinct from the loci for sugar and amino acid transport.[236]

End-products of nitrogen metabolism.   Knowledge of the intermediary nitrogen metabolism of cestodes is fragmentary.   Although the nitrogenous compounds excreted by a number of species of cestodes have been examined, the metabolic pathways whereby these end-products are produced are almost unknown.   The major end-products appear to be urea, uric acid and ammonia, although a remarkable array of

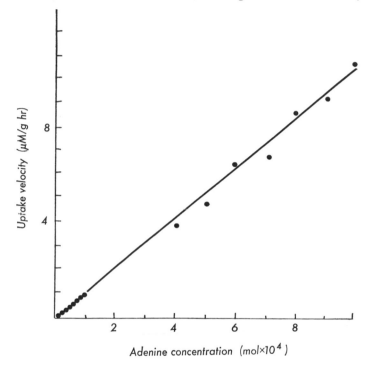

FIG. 31. Uptake of adenine in *Hymenolepis diminuta*.   Note that lack of saturation indicates entry by diffusion over concentration range tested.   (After MacInnis, *et al.*, 1965.)

other nitrogen-containing compounds have been detected (Table 27). Few quantitative estimations of the relative importance of the major end-products have been made.   In the case of *H. diminuta*, 2–10 times more ammonia than urea is produced (Table 28).[53]   It is generally held that ammonotelic organisms live in habitats where water is freely available to remove end-products, whereas ureotelic organisms usually occur in environments where they have to economise with water usage. Although parasitic helminths are thought to be ammonotelic, the rate of synthesis of urea by *H. diminuta*[53] is about 1 mg per g worms (w.w.)

per day (o·7 μ mole/g worm/hr) which is well within the range reported for ureotelic vertebrates. It must be stressed, however, that the terms 'ammonotelic' and 'ureotelic' should be used with caution; they are essentially relative terms, and the limits of their usage need defining to be of any real value.

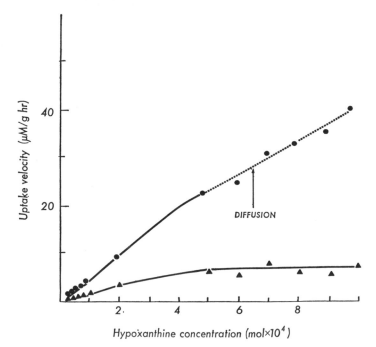

FIG. 32. Uptake of hypoxanthine by *Hymenolepis diminuta*. The upper curve represents observed values; dashed portion represents slope (=33·33) used as diffusion rate. The lower curve represents total uptake minus the diffusion component. The area below the lower curve thus is considered as mediated transport; points are means of four samples. (After MacInnis, *et al.*, 1965.)

Ammonia can be produced metabolically by a number of different enzymes, such as amino acid oxidase. An amino acid oxidase, active with L-glutamic acid, has been reported in *H. diminuta*.[87] Ammonia may also be obtained via urease, an enzyme reported in the trypanorhynchids, *Lacistorhynchus tenuis* and *Pterobothrium lintoni*,[391] but the enzyme could not be detected in *Moniezia expansa*, *Taenia pisiformis*,[36] nor in tetraphyllidean cestodes[391] or the trypanorhynchid cestode *Grillotia erinaceus*.[391]

TABLE 26

Transaminase activity in three species of Hymenolepis.

Values are given in micromoles of amino acid/mg. N/hour. A zero value indicates that transminase activity could not be detected. (Data from Wertheim, et al.[477])

Amino donor	transaminase α-ketoglutaric→ glutamic			transaminase pyruvic→ alanine		
	H. diminuta	*H. citelli*	*H. nana*	*H. diminuta*	*H. citelli*	*H. nana*
Alanine	5·0	4·5	0	—	—	—
Aspartic acid	17·7	28·6	31·9	3·1	0	0
Asparagine	3·8	4·0	3·8	0·9	0	0
Glutamic acid	—	—	—	13·4	14·1	8·5

Production of urea by cestodes suggests the existence of a (Krebs-Henseleit) ornithine cycle, the basic pathway of which is shown in Fig. 34. Two important enzymes of the ornithine cycle, arginase and

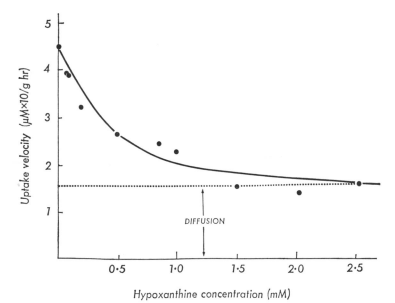

FIG. 33. Effect of increasing hypoxanthine concentration on the uptake of 0·02mM uracil by *Hymenolepis diminuta*. The degree of uptake which could not be inhibited by the highest concentrations of hypoxanthine is considered to represent entry by diffusion. (After MacInnis *et al.*, 1965.)

ornithine transcarbamylase have been identified in cestodes. Arginase has been detected in a number of cyclophyllidean species: *Moniezia benedeni*, *Taenia pisiformis*[36] and *Hymenolepis* spp.,[53, 55]—in addition to some tetraphyllidean and trypanorhynchid cestodes of elasmobranchs.

TABLE 27

Nitrogen excretory products of cestodes

Excretory Product	H. diminuta (Fairbairn, et al.[101] ; Campbell[153])	*E. granulosus (von Brand[36]: Krvavica, et al.[208])	*Cysticercus tenuicollis (von Brand[36])	Lacistorhynchus tenuis (Simmons[391])	*Hydatigera taeniaeformis (Haskins & Olivier[145])
Ammonia	+	−	−	+	+
Urea	+	+	+	−	+
Uric acid	−	+	+	−	−
Methylamine	−	−	−	−	+
Ethylamine	−	−	−	−	+
Propylamine	−	−	−	−	−
Butylamine	−	−	−	−	+
Amylamine	−	−	−	−	−
Heptylamine	−	−	−	−	−
Ethylene diamine	−	−	−	−	+
Cadaverine	−	−	−	−	+
Ethanolamine	−	−	−	−	−
1-amino-2-propanol	−	−	−	−	+
Amino acids	?	+	−	−	+
Creatinine	−	+	+	−	−
Betaine	−	+	−	−	−

* larva

Ornithine transcarbamylase has also been detected in many of these species, with the exception of the tetraphyllid *Phyllobothrium foliatum*.[55] The properties of arginase have been examined in detail[53] and it has been shown to have a dependence on Mn^{2+} and Co^{2+} ions and a sharp pH optimum at 9·5.

The occurrence of these enzymes, together with the demonstration that $^{14}CO_2$ was incorporated into urea, provides evidence for the operation of the ornithine cycle in *H. diminuta*. However, a *functional* ornithine cycle has not been detected in *M. expansa*, *D. caninum*, *T. pisiformis* and *E. granulosus* despite the presence of ornithine transcarbamylase and arginase in these species.[180a] In no case was carbamyl phosphate synthetase detectable. It has been suggested that those enzymes of the ornithine cycle which were present might be concerned in metabolic activities other than the synthesis of urea.[180a]

In addition to the more normal excretory products of nitrogen metabolism, a number of cestodes have been shown to excrete amino acids e.g. *H. taeniaeformis* larva[145], *E. granulosus*,[208] and *A. magna*.[207]

TABLE 28

Formation of ammonia and urea by Hymenolepis diminuta in vitro, *during incubation in balanced saline for 1 hour at 38°C*
(Data from Campbell[53])

Flask additions (12 μ mole)	μmole urea/g/hr		μmole NH$_3$/g/hr
	Colorimetric method	Enzymatic method	2
None	0·69	0·51	1·32
None (minus antibiotics)	0·71	0·69	1·05
L-arginine	2·43	2·32	1·92
L-citrulline	—	0·80	0·88
L-ornithine	0·59	0·39	1·55
L-aspartate	0·78	0·84	8·49
L-alanine	0·89	0·78	2·03
L-glutamate	0·85	0·72	1·12
L-glutamine	0·99	—	—

The significance of this phenomenon is not, at present, clear. Many experiments on excretion are carried out under abnormal conditions

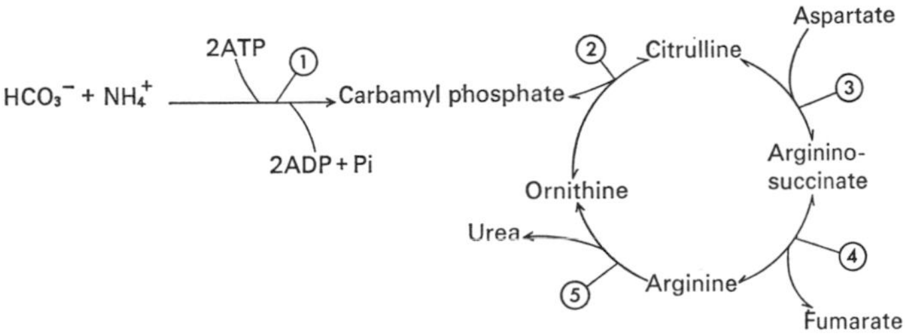

FIG. 34. The (Krebs-Henseleit) ornithine cycle. Numbers refer to enzymes as follows: (1) Carbamyl phosphate synthetase (E.C.2.7.2.a). (2) Ornithine transcarbamylase (E.C.2.1.3.3). (3) Arginino succinate synthetase (E.C.6.3.4.5). (4) Arginino succinate lyase (E.C.4.3.2.1). (5) Arginase (E.C.3.5.3.1).

and the release of amino acids may merely represent 'abnormal' leakage from the tissues. Excretion of amino acids has also been reported from trematodes and nematodes.

Lipid Metabolism

General Considerations

The lipid metabolism of cestodes has been examined to only a limited extent, and most studies have been confined to quantitative and qualitative examination of the lipid content and its distribution in the tissues. Although these studies cover a number of species (Table 29), the introduction of new methods of lipid analysis, such as gas, column and thin layer chromotography and infrared and ultraviolet spectroscopy, has so revolutionised this field, that the results of work carried out earlier than about 1960 must be accepted with some reservation. For this reason, only the results of the most recent work are discussed here. For the early work see the reviews of von Brand,[34, 36] Read and Simmons[316] and Smyth.[406]

The role of lipids in cestode metabolism is not clear. There is no evidence, for example, that lipids act as energy reserves in cestodes, as they do in nematodes. Furthermore, the synthesis of lipids appears to have been studied only in *H. diminuta*.[120] In this species only a limited capacity for fatty acid biosynthesis has been demonstrated and most of its fatty acids appear to be derived from the host. Although most of the incorporated label from ^{14}C-starch appeared in glycogen or excretory products, significant amounts appeared in phospholipids. Also, some fatty acid synthesis occurred from 1-^{14}C-palmitate and 1-^{14}C-acetate.[120]

Lipid Analyses

Quantitative. Lipids can be divided broadly into simple lipids, comprising the fats (triglycerol esters of fatty acids), waxes (esters of fatty acids with complex monohydric alcohols), and compound lipids, comprising the phospholipids and the glycolipids. Steroids are also included in the latter group. In vertebrates the steroids include substances such as cholesterol, bile acids, sex and other metabolic hormones.

The relative amounts of lipids reported in cestodes are given in Table 9, from which it is clear that there is considerable variation from species to species. Moreover, the lipid content of some species grown in different hosts may vary substantially. Thus, *H. diminuta* from hamsters contained 9·5% lipid (d.w.) and those from Long-Evans rats 16·5% (d.w.).[472] A further factor must also be taken into account when analysis figures are being considered, namely the degree of maturity of the proglottids, for it has been shown[101] that in *H. diminuta* lipids tend to be more abundant in the most posterior proglottids.

Figures for ' total lipids ' thus tend to be somewhat meaningless unless the degree of maturity is known.

The higher content of lipid in older proglottids has led to the view that much of this lipid largely represents waste products of metabolism.[34, 36] This is an attractive hypothesis, for higher fatty acids are known to be by-products of carbohydrate metabolism (Chapter 5). Yet, in *H. diminuta*, the experimental evidence is against this view; for appreciable numbers of carbon atoms absorbed are not incorporated into fatty acids.[120]

TABLE 29

Phospholipids identified in cestodes
(Data from von Brand[36] ; Harrington[143])

(+ = present   o = absent   tr = trace   — = no information)

Species	Cephalins	Lecithins	Inositol phosphatides	Sphingomyelin	Cardiolipin	Plasmalogens
Diphyllobothrium latum	+	+	—	—	—	—
Echinococcus granulosus	—	+	—	—	—	—
Hymenolepis diminuta	+	+	+	tr	+	+
Hymenolepis citelli	+	+	+	tr	+	+
Taenia saginata	—	+	+	—	—	—
Hydatigera taeniaeformis	+	+	o	+	—	—

Qualitative. One of the more unusual features of the composition of cestode lipids is the fact that unsaponifiable material and phospholipids often account for more than 20% of the total lipids.[36, 101, 237]

The unsaponifiable fraction is largely cholesterol, accompanied by other sterol-like materials in some cases. Cholesterol, has been identified in *T. saginata*[76], *H. diminuta*,[101] *Hydatigera taeniaeformis*,[453] *M. expansa*,[453] *D. latum*,[316] and *E. granulosus*.[74] In the last two species, cholesterol amounted to 98% and 85% respectively, of the unsaponifiable material.[453]

Glycolipids (cerebrosides and gangliosides) in higher vertebrates typically occur in the nervous system. They have been reported in *M. expansa*, *H. taeniaeformis*, *D. latum*,[36] *H. diminuta*[101], and *H. citelli*,[143] and in some cases at levels which suggest that they are not confined to the rather simple nervous system of cestodes.

A number of studies on the fatty acids bound to glycerol, sterols and phospholipids have been made on cestodes. However, the introduction of gas chromatography to a study of the fatty acids in other parasitic groups (especially protozoa) suggests that much of the early work on cestodes[34, 36] will need re-examination by this method. Column chromatography has also revolutionised lipid analyses.

For example, early analysis (by paper chromatography) of saturated fatty acids of *T. saginata*[76] revealed only the presence of palmitic and stearic acid, whereas application of advanced chromatographic methods[235] further revealed the presence of arachidic, myristic, lauric acids and oleo-palmitic (unsat.). Detailed analyses of the lipids of *H. citelli* and *H. diminuta* by modern chromatographic methods are available.[119, 143]

Incorporation of fatty acids. Studies with labelled compounds have shown that *H. diminuta* is permeable to acids such as acetate, stearate, palmitate, oleate and linoleate.[180, 231a] This species moreover appears to have lost its capacity for *de novo* synthesis of fatty acids, and these substances must therefore be absorbed from the host intestinal contents. The inability to synthesise fatty acids may be related to the anaerobic environment of the gut[180] Acetate carbon, unlike fatty acid carbon, is incorporated primarily with phospholipids and probably with saturated and unsaturated acids.

Enzymes. Since the introduction of histochemical methods for esterases and cholinesterases, some studies on the distribution of these have been carried out in cestodes; these have been dealt with earlier (p. 19). The (non-specific) indoxylacetate technique and the (specific) acetylthiocholine iodide technique (p. 19), for example, beautifully demonstrate cholinesterase in the nervous system (Plate I); this substance has also been detected by chemical means (p. 22). Concentrations of non-specific esterases have also been reported in the tegument in some species (Table 2). The significance of this is not clear, but it may indicate the ability of the tegument to break down lipids at the host/parasite interface, although there is no direct evidence as yet that such a process does occur.

APPENDIX

Active Transport

Theoretical Considerations

The mechanisms involved in active transport are not understood, although a number of hypotheses have been postulated. These are basically similar in two respects. Firstly, they postulate that the absorbed material must be transported by a ' carrier ', and secondly, that the separating membrane is ' asymmetric ', i.e. materials can be transported only one way. This latter process could be explained if we postulated the existence of two different enzymes, located at the outer edge of the membrane, which catalyse different reactions. The absorbed substance A would react with substance B under the influence of enzyme E_1 to produce an end-product AB which in turn would react with enzyme E_2 to produce end-product A—a proposed scheme which would allow the carrier solute complex to move with a gradient in the membrane.

Studies on active transport have shown that the relationship between the velocity of uptake of a substance and its concentration follows the well-known Michaelis-Menten equation of classical enzyme kinetics (sometimes known as ' saturation ' kinetics). This *suggests* that enzyme systems are involved in active transport, but it is stressed that mathematical similarities cannot be regarded as proof that similar mechanisms operate: they are more likely to indicate the same kind of surface-contact saturation phenomenon.

In an enzyme-substrate reaction, we are dealing with a reaction in which, over a certain concentration, a maximum velocity V_{max} is reached. In active transport, the same kind of quantitative relationship between absorption of a substance and concentration occurs. This relationship is expressed by the Michaelis-Menten equation:

$$V = \frac{V_{max}\, S}{K_m + S} \quad \text{or} \quad K_m = S\left(\frac{V_{max}}{V} - 1\right) \quad \text{or} \quad V = \frac{V_{max}}{1 + \dfrac{K_m}{S}}$$

where V = velocity or reaction
V_{max} = maximum velocity of reaction
K_m = Michaelis constant (essentially the dissociation constant of the enzyme-substrate complex)
S = substrate concentration.

This equation is derived as in the following manner.

Consider an enzyme E reacting with substrate S to form an enzyme-substrate complex $E\!:\!S$ which in turn releases the product P, thus

$$E + S \underset{k_2}{\overset{k_1}{\rightleftharpoons}} E\!:\!S \xrightarrow{\;k_3\;} P + E$$

Let e = the concentration of total enzyme and c the concentration of enzyme-substrate complex.

Applying the law of mass action the velocity (V_1) of formation of $E\!:\!S$ is proportional to the concentration of the reactants

$$V_1 = k_1\,(e - c)S$$

and the velocity of the reverse reaction V_2 is

$$V_2 = k_2 c$$

at equilibrium $V_1 = V_2$ and $k_1 (e-c)S = k_2 c$

$$\text{Therefore} \quad \frac{(e-c)S}{c} = \frac{k_2}{k_1} = K_m$$

$$\frac{eS}{c} - S = K_m \quad \text{or} \quad c = \frac{eS}{K_m + S}$$

The overall velocity V is assumed to be governed by the rate of breakdown of the enzyme-substrate complex c, and therefore, the rate of formation of c is in excess of the rate of decomposition and hence $k_1 > k_2 \gg k_3$; the decomposition of the enzyme-substrate complex is the rate determining step :

$$\text{Therefore} \quad V = k_3 c$$

and, substituting in the equation above,

$$V = \frac{k_3 e S}{K_m + S}$$

When $V = V_{max}$, i.e. is the maximum rate of reaction, then all the enzyme is in the form of enzyme-substrate complex and the reaction is of zero order with respect to substrate and $V_{max} = k_3 e$, so that

$$V = \frac{V_{max} \, S}{K_m + S}$$

which is one form of the Michaelis-Menten equation, as above. The equation can also be expressed as

$$\frac{1}{V} = \frac{K_m + S}{V_{max} \, S} = \frac{K_m}{V_{max}} \cdot \frac{1}{S} + \frac{1}{V_{max}}$$

and a reaction following this equation should give a straight line when $1/V$ is plotted against $1/S$ (a Lineweaver-Burk reciprocal plot) (Fig. 29), whereas V plotted against S is, of course, non-linear.

In the application of these equations to the demonstration of active transport of materials into cells the notation K_t is sometimes used to represent a ' transport ' constant instead of the Michaelis constant K_m.

7: The Biology of the Egg

General Account

Many of the activities of cestodes are directed towards egg-production, and thus for an understanding of the physiology and biochemistry of the group it is important to have information on the structure, chemical composition and mode of formation of the egg. For example, in some cyclophyllids the embryophore consists of keratin,[184, 249, 283] and maturing worms may therefore be expected to have a major nutritional requirement for keratin precursors. In contrast, the pseudophyllid egg has a sclerotin capsule (p. 111), for which different precursors will be necessary.

The cestode egg particularly lends itself to studies on such topics as (*a*) the histochemistry and biochemistry of the structural proteins mentioned above, (*b*) the ultrastructure of embryonic membranes, (*c*) the physiology of ' hatching ' and the role of enzymes, biochemical or biophysical stimuli in this process, and (*d*) the physiology of ' activation ' of hatched oncospheres.

The Formation of the Egg

Anatomy of Reproductive System

Female. As has been stressed, the form of the egg in each cestode class is closely correlated to the structure of the female genitalia. The most important point of variation occurs in the vitellaria, which in some orders (Pseudophyllidea, Trypanorhyncha, Tetraphyllidea and Proteocephaloidea) are extensive and synthesise in their vitelline cells both yolk and egg-shell; in this respect they show a striking homology with the Trematoda. In other groups (especially the Cyclophyllidea) the vitellaria are small and are concerned largely with the production of yolk material (Fig. 38). This question is considered further below (pp. 109-115).

Male. The male system, which is based on the typical platyhelminth plan, presents no unusual features. The testes may be in small dispersed groups (e.g. *Taenia*) or in large well-formed bodies (e.g. *Hymenolepis*). Cestode spermatogenesis, which has been reviewed in detail,[350] shows no unusual features except that the number of spermatozoa in a morula is 64 in contrast with that in trematodes where it is 32.

A number of studies on the histochemistry and ultrastructure of cestode spermatozoa have been made. Although these show some differences from trematodes and other invertebrates, none of these differences appears to be obviously related to physiological differences.

The histochemistry of spermatozoa in the following species has been investigated:

Triaenophorus lucii,[347] *Baerietta diana* and *Distoichometra kozloffi*,[94] *Dipylidium caninum*[348, 349] and *Taenia saginata*.[279] Ultrastructure studies have been made on *Proteocephalus pollanicola*,[135] *H. nana* and *H. diminuta*.[226, 336]

Although the cross section of a sperm tail reveals the typical flagellum arrangement of nine peripheral and two central filaments, the latter differ from the typical pattern in that one of the central filaments is enclosed by the other and in longitudinal section the outer filament appears to form a helix round the central filament.[336]

Insemination and Fertilisation

The physiology of the insemination process is not known; which is not surprising considering the extreme difficulty of studying this process. There is no information as to whether an internal, sexual endocrine system exists or a sexual chemotactic attraction occurs. Both self-impregnation within the same proglottid and impregnation of an adjacent proglottid of the same strobila, or impregnation of a proglottid of a different strobila, are believed to occur. At least in some species, compression of a strobila against the gut wall is a necessary prerequisite for copulation and impregnation to occur. This may be readily demonstrated experimentally with *Schistocephalus solidus*. When this species is matured *in vitro* under compression within a narrow cellulose tube (Fig. 68), impregnation occurs, the *receptaculum seminis* contains spermatozoa and fertile eggs are produced.[410] In contrast, worms matured within the same culture vessel but *outside* the tube have empty receptacula and produce only infertile eggs. From this it is assumed that compression either (*a*) allows the cirrus to be bent around into the vaginal pore of the same or an adjacent proglottid, or (*b*) permits a concentration of spermatozoa to be built up in a confined space and hence more readily drawn into the vagina.

Fertilisation has been described in a number of species[350] but it appears that nothing is known of the physiology of the process.

Types of Cestode Eggs

Physiological studies on cestode eggs have been confined largely to the pseudophyllid and cyclophyllid egg (Fig. 35), undoubtedly

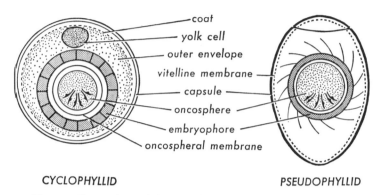

CYCLOPHYLLID   PSEUDOPHYLLID

FIG. 35. Comparison of the morphology of a cyclophyllidean and a pseudophyllidean egg. (After Smyth, 1963.)

because the most easily obtained cestode species occur in these groups. The formation of the capsule or egg-shell (p. 108) has been extensively investigated—especially in a series of detailed studies by Löser[222-4]— and these processes are dealt with in detail below. It is worthwhile, however, to survey all the types of cestode eggs which occur, so that an overall picture can be obtained. The field has been the subject of a number of reviews.[72, 222-4, 350, 417, 424]

Formation of the Embryonic Envelopes

A fully formed egg is enclosed in a number of membranes, some of which harden to produce protective ' envelopes '. Although the word 'envelope' is widely used (and is used here) it is not perhaps an entirely appropriate word for these structures. It has a common connotation implying a *thin* covering layer, whereas some of the egg ' envelopes ' are relatively thick. It is important for the study of the penetration of substances into the egg, as well as for understanding the physiology of hatching, that the origin and nature of these envelopes be understood. Rybicka[350] has provided a valuable review of this field, and her terminology is followed below. The main confusion has arisen from the fact that although there are only four *primary* embryonic envelopes, some of these give rise to secondary structures, so that more than this number may be found in a fully formed egg. The four embryonic envelopes are as follows:

The capsule is well developed in the Pseudophyllidea, Tetraphyllidea and Trypanorhyncha, where it forms a strong, waterproof covering; it is generally poorly developed or absent in Cyclophyllidea.

The outer envelope—formed from two or three macromeres—becomes hardened in some species; in Cyclophyllidea it divides, to give a ' coat ', and an ' outer envelope '.[350]

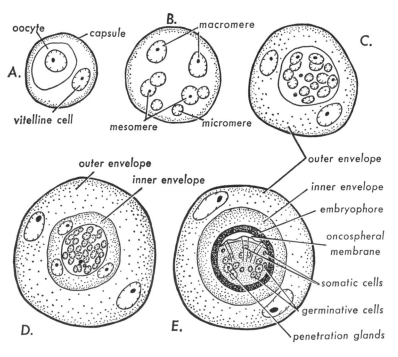

FIG. 36. Embryonic development in the Cyclophyllidea; diagrammatic. A. fertilised oocyte; B. cleaving embryo; C. early preoncosphere; D. late preoncosphere; E. oncosphere. (After Rybicka, 1964.)

The inner envelope. The origin of this envelope, which arises later than the other two, is obscure. Part of this structure gives rise to the embryophore (Fig. 36E; pp. 114-115).

The oncospheral membrane. This is a thin membrane, of unknown origin, which lies beneath the embryophore and surrounds the oncosphere (Fig. 36E). It is of considerable physiological importance, as it serves as a barrier to penetrating substances.

There appear to be four main types of cestode eggs,[222] the formation of which is summarised in Fig. 38. These may be broadly grouped together into two groups:

Group I. The Pseudophyllidea-type egg. Eggs with a thick sclerotin (p. 112) capsule, produced by cestodes with well-developed vitellaria, i.e. Pseudophyllidea, Trypanorhyncha and Tetraphyllidea. The cestodes in this group generally infect aquatic (rather than terrestrial) hosts; their life cycles are normally associated with water, in which

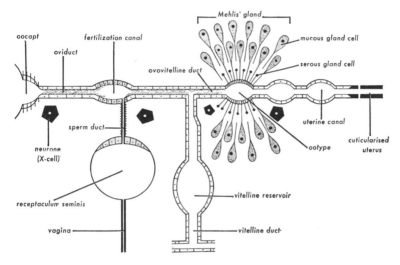

FIG. 37. Schematic representation of the egg-forming apparatus (=Oogenotop) of a pseudophyllidean cestode. (After Löser, 1965a.)

the egg embryonates and into which a coracidium hatches; the hatched larva is then ingested by the first aquatic intermediate host. This type of egg is homologous with the trematode egg.[422] More rarely (e.g. *Archigetes*), the egg hatches only when ingested by the intermediate host (p. 119).

Group II. Remaining egg types. The eggs in this group are generally embryonated when laid, and do not normally require a free-living aquatic stage in the life cycle. Although most of the well-known species have a terrestrial intermediate host, usually an arthropod or a vertebrate, many species have aquatic intermediate hosts,[181] e.g. *Aploparaksis furcigera* (in oligochaetes); *Dicranotaenia coronula* (in copepods); *Diorchis ransomi* (in ostracods); *Echinocotyle rosseteri* (in molluscs). The size, shape, and even the density, of the eggs in this group represent

adaptations to the life cycle and biotope of the intermediate host.[181]
Eggs are often heavy, such as the eggs of *Hymenolepis megalops*, which
are eaten by the benthic ostracod *Cypris pubera*. In contrast, some eggs
float, such as those of *Hymenolepis furcifera*, which are accessible to

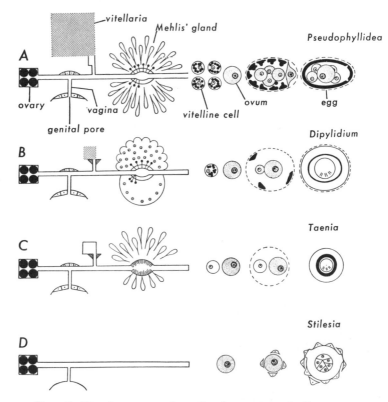

FIG. 38. The four types of egg-forming systems (=Oogenotop,
p. 112) in cestodes. A. Cestodaria, Pseudophyllidea, Trypanorhyncha, Tetraphyllidea. B. Some Cyclophyllidea, e.g. *Dipylidium*.
C. Taeniidae, e.g. *Taenia*. D. Thysanosominae, e.g. *Stilesia*.
For explanation see text. (After Löser, 1965b.)

swimming copepods and ostracods.[181] An extraordinarily specialised
and unusual morphological adaptation is found in *Diorchis stefańskii*,
in which the embryophore is delicately striped, resembling the diatoms
on which the intermediate host, *Dolerocypris fasciata*, feeds.[181]

Three types of eggs are found in Group II.

(i) The *Dipylidium-type* egg (Fig. 38B) with a thin capsule (p. 108) and relatively thin embryophore; embryonated when laid, e.g. *Dipylidium, Moniezia, Hymenolepis*.

(ii) The *Taenia-type* egg (Fig. 38C) lacking an outer sclerotin capsule but often covered with a very delicate membrane (which is normally not seen in faecal eggs); the embryophore is very thick and striated, e.g. *Taenia, Hydatigera, Echinococcus*.

(iii) The *Stilesia-type* egg (Fig. 38D) formed from genitalia in which vitellaria are lacking, so that the egg is formed only from the components of the egg and sperm. The uterus wall, however, lays down a thick cellular covering, e.g. *Stilesia, Avitellina*. Formation of the main types of eggs is further considered below.

Formation of the Pseudophyllidea-type Egg

General mechanism. It has been pointed out that this type of egg is formed in a manner almost identical to that which takes place in trematodes.[422] This is not surprising; for the female genitalia in the Pseudophyllidea and the Proteocephaloidea show striking homologies with the genitalia in trematodes. Investigation has largely centred around the formation of the egg-shell (capsule) and the biochemistry of the processes involved.

Species examined include: *Amphiptyches urna* (Gyrocotylidea), *Bothridium pithonis, Khawia iowensis, Caryophyllaeus laticeps, Eutetrarhynchus ruficollis, Triaenophorus nodulosus*,[222] *Echeneibothrium maculatum*;[222, 484] *D. latum*;[33, 222, 223] *Schistocephalus solidus*;[413] and *Proteocephalus filicollis*.[164]

The mechanism (Figs. 37, 38A) whereby this type of egg, with its sclerotin capsule, is formed appears to be similar in all the above species, with some minor variations, and may be summarised as follows:

Ova are released periodically from the ovary and pass down the oviduct to the ootype where fertilisation takes place; a sphincter muscle controls the release of ova. Mature vitelline cells, which contain both shell and yolk precursors, pass from the vitelline glands to the vitelline reservoir, where they may be temporarily stored. Vitelline cells pass from the reservoir to the ootype and in this region release the globules of shell-precursor which coalesce to form a capsule. The secretion of Mehlis' gland, which is more fully discussed below, may play a part in this release, and it has been suggested that one of its secretions (from the serous glands) has surface-active action.[223] Another secretion (from the mucous glands) is believed to form a ground lamella for the capsule (p. 108). The capsule, which is unhardened at this stage thus encloses both the ovum and the remains of the vitelline cells—the latter serving as yolk reserves (= ' true ' yolk) for the fully formed egg. The shape of the ootype appears to determine the shape of the finished egg.[223] As the eggs pass along the uterus, and out through the uterine pore, the protein of the shell becomes tanned by the quinone formed during the process (p. 113) and the eggs may visibly darken in colour. Due to the bonding of the protein chains by quinone (Fig. 40), the protein egg-shell becomes stabilised and hardened and loses its affinity for protein stains. The operculum appears to be formed by the action of the ovum, which sends out two fine pseudopodia-like extensions (Fig. 38A), which cause weakening at their point of contact with the hardening shell.[222] Nerve ganglia associated with this system, presumably co-ordinate the egg producing mechanisms. Löser[222] has coined the word 'Oogenotop' to describe the whole co-ordinated apparatus involved in egg formation (Fig. 37).

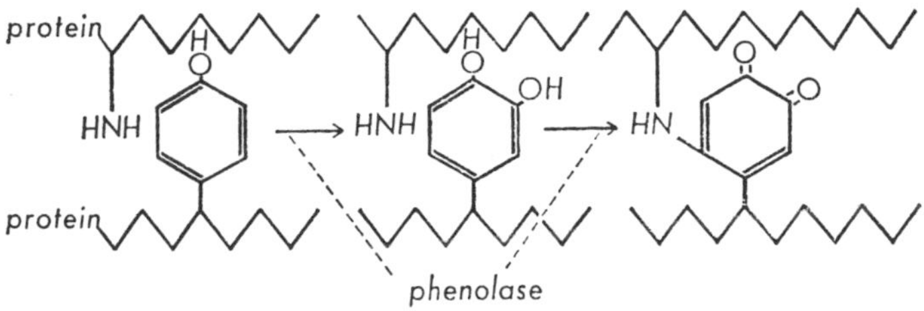

tyrosine *dopa* *dopa-quinone reacts with free NH_2 groups*

FIG. 39. Chemical reactions involved in quinone tanning. (After Smyth, 1966.)

Chemistry of quinone tanning in the pseudophyllid-type egg. The egg-shell (= capsule) in a number of pseudophyllid-type eggs has been shown to consist of a highly resistant type of protein, termed *sclerotin*.[33, 72, 222–3, 413, 424] This is a 'tanned protein' and one which occurs in widely divergent groups, in both invertebrates and vertebrates.[46] For example, the insect cuticle, the egg-cases of cockroaches and elasmobranchs and the byssus of the mussel *Mytilus*[411] consist chiefly of a sclerotin-type protein. The process of 'tanning', or sclerotinisation, is accomplished by means of an o-quinone derived enzymatically from an o-phenol in the presence of oxygen. The quinone is generally held to react with free NH_2 groups in adjacent protein chains to form strong covalent cross-links, which produce a stable protein (Figs. 39, 40); many aspects of sclerotin formation, however, are not understood.[46]

These reactions may be summarised as follows:

phenol $\xrightarrow{\text{phenolase}}$ quinone

'tanned' protein = sclerotin

protein $\longrightarrow$ protein

Since the bulk of the egg-shell material comes from shell-precursors or *presclerotin*[46] in the vitelline cells, these cells may be expected to give positive results with cytochemical tests for proteins, phenols and phenolase. Some of the tests for these, especially for phenols and

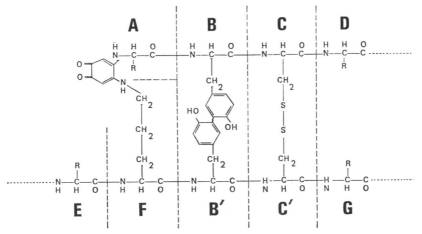

FIG. 40. Some of the covalent links that occur in proteins. ABCD represents one protein, EFB'C'G another. The N-terminal amino acid A is linked to an *o*-quinone which is also linked to a lysyl residue F (=quinone tanning); BB' represents two tyrosyl residues coupled by a biphenyl linkage; CC' represents two cysteinyl residues coupled by a cystine linkage (as in keratin); D, E and G are not cross-linked. (After Brünet, 1967.)

phenolase, give brightly coloured end-products and, when applied to whole worms, enable the vitellaria and eggs to be selectively stained in a remarkable manner. In general, however, the reactions—especially for phenols—are weaker in cestodes than in trematodes.[185] In some species, the vitellaria are not positive for phenolase so that some alternative tanning system may be present. For example, in the tetrarhynchs, *Gilquinia squali* and *Nybelina* sp., the vitellaria give some positive reactions for basic protein and phenols, but phenolase is present only in the latter.[328]

Although the phenolases in several species of trematodes have been isolated and their properties examined,[422] this has not yet been done for cestodes; neither have the phenolic materials been identified. To do so is likely to prove difficult; for even in insects—where much more material is available—the identification has taken many years. In the blowfly larva, *Calliphora*, for example, on which much work has been done, it has been demonstrated that labelled tyrosine, injected into a larva just before pupation, is converted into n-acetyldopamine which

$$
\begin{array}{l}
\text{HO—} \\
\text{HO—}
\end{array}
\bigcirc
\begin{array}{l}
\text{CH}_2\text{—CH}_2 \\
| \\
\text{HN—COCH}_3
\end{array}
$$

is then oxidised enzymatically to a quinone. In trematodes, a process of ' autotanning '[72] is possible, i.e. tanning may occur by the oxidation of the tyrosine bound to a protein, as above, since the vitelline globules of *Fasciola* have been shown to be rich in tyrosine; in contrast, the vitelline globules of *Diphyllobothrium latum* appear to be rich in histidine.[33]

Formation of the Dipylidium-*type egg*

This type of egg is characteristic of the Cyclophyllidea with the exception of the Taeniidae and the Thysanosominae; it also occurs in the Ichthyotaeniidea. It possesses only a thin capsule which appears to have its origin as a globule in the single yolk cell which takes part in the formation of the egg (Fig. 38B).

The nature of the outer capsule of eggs in this group (e.g. *Dipylidium*) has not been determined. On the basis of staining reaction, it has been stated[222-3] that this capsule is composed of sclerotin. Since the only unequivocal evidence for sclerotin is to demonstrate the existence of *all* the components of the quinone-tanning system—protein, phenol *and* the enzyme, phenolase, this result clearly requires confirmation by more rigorous techniques. Ultrastructure studies on *Dipylidium* have not provided any further evidence on the nature of the capsule.[283] In *Dipylidium*, 21 serous and 208 mucous gland cells are found in Mehlis' gland; in addition, apocrine gland cells occur in the uterus wall. The embryophore is not as thick as in the *Taenia*-type egg, but appears to be formed in the same way, *viz.* by the peripheral cells of the embryo, whose nuclei flatten and degenerate.[349] Like the taeniid embryophore, it appears to be keratin.[283]

Formation of the Taenia-*type Egg* (Fig. 38C)

This type of egg is formed in essentially the same way as that of the previous group; only one vitelline cell becomes associated with a fertilised ovum.[222-3] The vitelline cell lacks sclerotin precursors and no sclerotinised capsule is formed. The egg is wrapped in a thin membrane which is almost invisible in the recently laid egg and normally lost in faecal eggs. The embryophore in the *Taenia*-type egg is well developed and made up of minute keratin blocks which give it a characteristically radially striated appearance (Fig. 35). It is formed from the inner envelope of the pre-oncosphere (Fig. 36).

TABLE 30

Type of gland cells in Mehlis' gland in relation to the type of egg formed
(Based on data from Löser[223] ; Pence[283])

Form of egg	Sclerotin capsule	Mehlis' gland cells	
		Mucous	Serous
1. *Pseudophyllid*-type	+	+	+
2. *Dipylidium*-type	?*	+	+
3. *Taenia*-type	−	+	−
4. *Stilesia*-type	−	−	−

* See text p. 114

Function of Mehlis' Gland

The role of Mehlis' gland in the platyhelminths has long been a puzzle to parasitologists. The gland was sometimes known as the ' shell gland ', as it was believed to form the entire shell. The studies considered above make it clear that the shell material comes chiefly from the vitellaria. What, then, is the function of Mehlis' gland?

It was found that Mehlis' gland in a pseudophyllidean,[413] a cyclophyllidean cestode[184] and a trematode[424] were strongly PAS-positive and appeared to be secreting a mucopolysaccharide. An extensive study by Löser[222-3] has shown that two kinds of gland cells can occur in Mehlis' gland—mucous and serous gland cells. According to this author, the mucous secretion forms a ground lamella which surrounds the ovum and vitelline cells and on which the shell substance is laid down or, in the Taeniidae, it forms the fine lamella on which the embryophore is formed. In *Penetrocephalus ganapatii* the secretion of Mehlis' gland gives positive reactions for phospholipid which would be consistent with its formation of a membrane.[294] In trematodes, a lipoprotein membrane on *both* sides of the egg-shell has been reported in *Fasciola*,[70-1] and a comparable situation may occur in pseudophyllids, although this remains to be demonstrated. The number of mucous gland cells appears to be closely correlated with the intensity of egg production, a result not inconsistent with its possible function outlined above; the higher the number of eggs in a proglottid, the greater the number of cells (Fig. 41).

Since the serous gland cells are lacking in the Taeniidae and the Thysanosominae, which do not form a sclerotin capsule, but are present in those species which do (Table 30), it has been conjectured that these glands may secrete a surface-active agent which assists in the running together of the (presclerotin?) globules.[223] This view, which

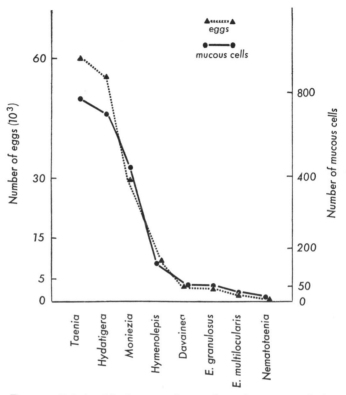

FIG. 41. Relationship between the number of mucous cells in Mehlis' gland and the number of formed eggs in a proglottid. (After Löser, 1965b.)

clearly requires confirmation by chemical means, is supported by the fact that the number of serous gland cells is highest in those species which form a thick capsule (Fig. 42).

Embryonation and Viability

The major studies on egg embryonation and viability have been carried out on pseudophyllid and cyclophyllid eggs.

Pseudophyllidean Eggs

Viability. These eggs normally require water for embryonation, and desiccation rapidly kills them. Survival and subsequent embryonation of the eggs of many species, after storage for several weeks, or

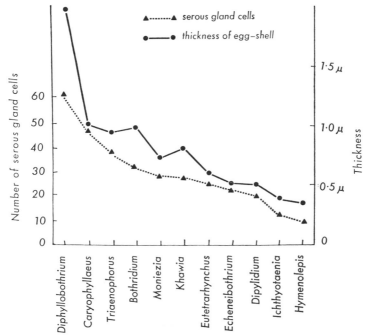

FIG. 42. Relationship between the number of serous cells in Mehlis' gland and the thickness of the egg-shell; this is known to be sclerotin in some cases. (After Löser, 1965b.)

even months, at refrigerator temperatures (2°– 4°C) has been described: e.g. *Spirometra mansonoides*,[253] *D. latum*,[137] *D. ursi* and *D. dalliae*,[158] *Triaenophorus lucii*.[136]

In contrast, the eggs of *Schistocephalus solidus* would not embryonate after only a 'short' period at this temperature. The lethal temperature of most pseudophyllidean eggs is probably about −5° to −8°C, and the eggs of *D. latum* are permanently damaged at this temperature, and cannot survive below −8°C.[138] The upper lethal temperature has been little studied; in *D. latum* it is above 30–35°C.[138] Even in embryonated eggs the mortality rate of coracidia before hatching may be extremely high. In *D. latum*, less than 75% of eggs from human hosts, and less than 1% of eggs from canine hosts, liberate coracidia,[187] although some workers have reported higher percentages.

Embryonation. It can be expected that as—with most invertebrate eggs—the physico-chemical factors which are known to influence biological reactions generally, will influence embryonation. Only the effect of temperature appears to have been examined to date; and the influence of other factors, especially pO_2, pCO_2, pH and E_h would make an interesting study.

Rather surprisingly, the embryos of pseudophyllids vary greatly in their response to temperature, an effect which has been termed 'thermal specificity'.[136] Such an effect, along with other factors of the biotope, could play an important role in determining the distribution of a species. For example, at 18–$20°C$ eggs of *D. latum* require 8–9 days' embryonation[138] and yet, at the same temperature, eggs of *T. lucii* require only 5 days.[136] Other embryonation times, at $20°C$, are:[158] *Diphyllobothrium dendriticum*, 6–8 days; *D. cordatum*, 5 days; *D. ditremum*, 9 days; *Schistocephalus solidus*, 14–16 days.

Embryonation at warm-blooded temperatures can induce abnormalities. Thus, eggs of *Spirometra mansonoides* and *S. solidus* when incubated at 37–$40°C$, produce abnormal coracidia.[257, 408] Since eggs of these species are released in warm-blooded hosts, it is likely that, within the host gut, premature embryonation normally is inhibited by lack of oxygen.

Cyclophyllidean Eggs

Since these eggs are generally embryonated when laid, the question of the effect of external factors on embryonation is not relevant. Apparently nothing is known of the factors influencing embryonation within a proglottid.

The few reports available suggest that eggs of cyclophyllids are remarkably resistant to temperature, but may be sensitive to low humidities.[215] Thus, eggs of *Echinococcus multilocularis* were found to be infective after 54 days at $-26°C$, or after 24 hours at $51°C$.[365] Relative humidities $<25\%$ are rapidly lethal to the eggs of *E. granulosus* —the embryophore apparently disintegrating.[215] Eggs of *E. granulosus* and *T. pisiformis* have also been shown to be viable after 2 weeks in concentrated formalin (40% formaldehyde).[150] Eggs of *T. saginata* have been found, after one month, to be viable at 29–$30°C$, but dead at $58°C$.[396] At air temperatures, eggs of this species survived (on hay) for about 22 days, but were not viable after 10 weeks.[419] The eggs of *Drepanidotaenia lanceolata*, whose intermediate host is a copepod, fell off rapidly in infectivity when stored in water, the maximum viability being about three weeks at 18–$24°C$.[202] The upper lethal temperature was about 33 °C ; and lack of oxygen was found to inhibit development.

Hatching

As was pointed out earlier (p. 105), the cestode egg provides an interesting model for certain kinds of biological studies—especially responses to physico-chemical factors such as light, temperature, pO_2, and enzyme action. It is clearly of survival value for a species if (a) hatching is inhibited by conditions within the definitive host so that it does not occur prematurely (but see *H. nana*, p. 3) and (b) that, where hatching takes place in water, it is stimulated by ecological conditions which are also favourable to the intermediate host. In the progenetic pseudophyllid, *Archigetes* sp., eggs hatch only on ingestion by the tubificid host,[189] so that presumably, in this case either the contained embryo is stimulated to secrete an enzyme which attacks the operculum seal or else the digestive juices of the host are effective in this respect.

TABLE 31

Effect of light on the hatching of the eggs of some pseudophyllidean cestodes

Species	Light requirement for hatching	Reference
Diphyllobothrium latum	essential	130
Diphyllobothrium ursi	not essential	158
Diphyllobothrium dendriticum (?)	essential	158
Diphyllobothrium dalliae	not essential	158
Diphyllobothrium oblongatum	essential	419
Schistocephalus solidus	essential	412
Spirometra mansonoides	essential	253
Triaenophorus lucii	not essential	136
Triaenophorus nodulosus	not essential	130
Bothriocephalus scorpii	essential	130

Pseudophyllidean Eggs

Influence of light intensity on hatching. In trematodes, there is evidence that opening of the operculum depends on the release by the larva, when fully developed, of an enzyme which is released under the influence of light and attacks the opercular seal.[422] A similar mechanism may operate in those pseudophyllidean cestodes whose eggs similarly hatch on exposure to light. Not all pseudophyllidean eggs require light for hatching, however, and presumably in those that do not (Table 31), release of the 'hatching' enzyme (if it occurs, see p. 122) is controlled by factors other than light.

The effect of intensity and wavelength of light on egg hatching have been examined experimentally only in the case of *D. latum*.[130] Hatching occurred within 1 min. after exposure to white light of an intensity of 1,000 lux (Fig. 43), and almost all eggs which were capable of hatching were hatched within 5–6 mins. The minimum light intensity which caused maximum percentage of hatching lay between

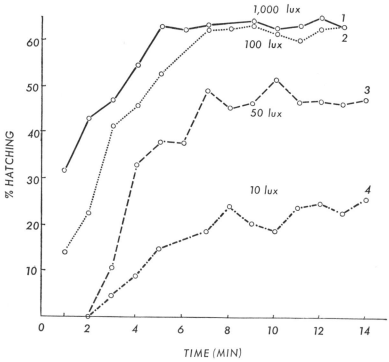

FIG. 43. Influence of intensity of light on the hatching of eggs of *Diphyllobothrium latum*. (After Grabiec, Guttowa & Michajlow, 1963a.)

50–100 lux acting for 30–60 seconds. Higher energy levels, acting for longer periods of time, failed to increase the percentage hatching. The minimal amount of energy for causing maximal hatching has been calculated to be 10^{-9} W per egg.

Influence on wavelength of light on hatching. Interesting experiments have been carried out to determine whether a particular wavelength, or range of wavelengths, stimulates maximum hatching of the embryonated eggs of *D. latum*.[130] The results of these experiments, which utilised four light-intensities—10, 50, 75 and 100 lux and exposure periods of 3 sec and 60 sec—are given in Table 32 and Fig. 44. There appear to be two peak values of hatching at wavelengths of about 300 mμ (ultraviolet) and 600 mμ (yellow). Infrared rays failed to initiate hatching, and in the red region light of 693 mμ to 704 mμ showed only a very weak stimulating effect.

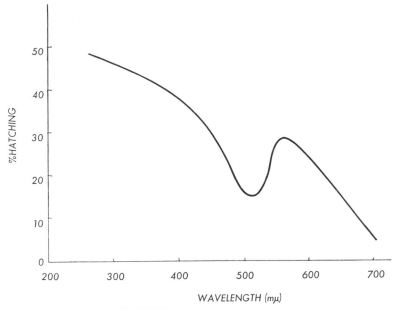

FIG. 44. Influence of wavelength of light on the hatching of the eggs of *Diphyllobothrium latum*; intensity 75 lux for 60 seconds. (After Grabiec, Guttowa & Michajlow, 1963a.)

Peaks of hatching in the yellow and ultraviolet bands approximately could possibly be explained on the grounds of light penetration in shallow and also deep water. Thus, limnological studies have shown that (a) yellow and green rays (500–600 mμ) penetrate farthest into deep water, and (b) ultraviolet light, although penetrating poorly into deep water, carries the greatest energy into shallow water.

Ecological implications of hatching mechanism. Since the eggs of *D. latum* tend to occur mostly in shallow water near the shores of closed water bodies, it can be assumed that they would normally be exposed to the peak wavelengths shown above. The hatching phenomenon may thus be regarded as an adaptation presumably related to the ecology of the copepod intermediate hosts. It can be speculated, for example, that under the influence of sunlight, a large number of eggs may hatch at once, and the same light intensity could be associated with a similar release of copepod larva, or a phototropic migration of intermediate hosts towards the area where the eggs are hatching. In contrast, the eggs of several other species, e.g. *Diphyllobothrium dalliae, D. ursi*,[158] *Triaenophorus nodulosus*,[130] are capable of hatching in the dark. This hatching behaviour undoubtedly has survival value; for these species have been found either in deep lakes or in muddy pools with suspended colloids. Some limited experiments have been carried out also on the effect of salinity on the hatching of pseudophyllid eggs.[158] On the

TABLE 32

Effect of wavelength on the hatching (%) *of the eggs of* Diphyllobothrium latum (Data from Grabiec, *et al.*[130])

Wave-length	3 sec.		60 sec.			Colour
	10 lux	50 lux	10 lux	75 lux	100 lux	
	o	o	o	o	o	infrared
704·0 mμ	o	3·2	o	13·3	13·4	red
693·0 mμ	o	3·6	o	12·0	16·4	red
595·0 mμ	20·0	–	6·7	33·3	34·4	yellow
576·0 mμ	28·7	21·0	9·5	31·1	30·3	yellow
547·5 mμ	22·4	24·2	10·0	32·5	38·5	yellow
530·0 mμ	17·1	21·8	7·0	29·2	23·8	green
448·0 mμ	23·6	32·9	10·3	39·1	41·7	violet
257·0 mμ	28·4	51·7	20·0	56·7	58·6	ultraviolet

basis of the degree of swelling at different osmotic pressures, species have been assigned to fresh-water, brackish-water or marine environments (Fig. 54).

Biochemistry of hatching. By analogy with trematodes (p. 119) it is likely that, under the influence of light, the fully developed embryo releases a 'hatching enzyme' which attacks a cement substance sealing the operculum. However, neither the existence of the cement substance nor of the enzyme has been demonstrated. The fact that hatching is stimulated by narrow bands of wavelengths suggest that a specific biochemical reaction is being activated. On theoretical grounds, this is likely to involve an enzyme; but confirmation of this hypothesis must await more detailed work.

Cyclophyllidean Eggs

Hatching of the cyclophyllidean egg involves two processes: (*a*) the passive digestion of the embryophore, (*b*) stimulation (= 'activation') of the hexacanth embryo to become motile and rupture its enclosing oncospheral membrane.[386]   These processes frequently require different stimuli for their initiation.

Hatching in Cyclophyllidea other than Taeniidae.   Hatching of the eggs of many species in this group have been reported to occur (sometimes at very low percentages) in very simple solutions, such as distilled water, physiological saline, or solutions containing various ions, especially Na^+ and Cl^-, e.g. *Dipylidium, Cittotaenia, Davainea,*[419] *Raillietina,*[326, 359, 362] *Hymenolepis.*[82]   In the natural intermediate host, hatching is probably brought about largely by the mechanical action of the mouth parts, a process undoubtedly assisted by the digestive secretions.   The hatching of the eggs in the Hymenolepididae has been extensively studied, and although techniques for hatching have been developed (see below), little precise information of the fundamental basis of the hatching mechanism is available.   In general, the process of hatching described in *H. diminuta,*[465] *H. microstoma, H. citelli* and *H. nana*[30, 30a, 366] differs only in detail.   Apparently the capsule is broken mechanically, and the vitelline layer digested by a substance or substances derived from the host gut; the oncosphere frees itself from its embryophore by its own activity.   In *Oochoristica vacuolata,* the embryophore, when in the gut of the arthropod host, becomes grooved internally in the plane of the lateral hooks of the oncosphere, thus indicating the extent of the mechanical action involved.[157]

In the natural host, the factors which stimulate oncosphere activity (= motility) are not clear.   In the case of *H. microstoma,* activity has been shown to be markedly stimulated by change in temperature, an effect possibly related to conditions in the intermediate host, the flour beetle *Tribolium,* whose temperature fluctuates from day to night.[82] Artificial methods developed for ' hatching ' the eggs of the various *Hymenolepis* species show some variation.[30, 30a]   In these, the capsule (= shell) is removed by mechanical agitation with glass beads and the effects of various enzymes, gas phases, etc. examined.   Since the capsule has been removed artificially, the term ' hatching ' is a slight misnomer and ' oncosphere release ' would be more appropriate for these experiments.

In *Hymenolepis* spp., oncosphere activation was related to the presence of dissociated $NaHCO_3$ and free CO_2, and enzyme action was essential;[30a] the pH was also important.   Trypsin was the most effective enzyme in bringing about optimal hatching, and α-amylase was found to dissolve the oncosphere coat of *H. diminuta*[30a].   Bile salts were not found necessary for hatching and were inhibitory in the case of *H. citelli* and *H. microstoma.*   Some experiments suggested that urea was essential for hatching of *H. nana,*[30] but this result was not confirmed by later work.[30a]

Hatching in the Taeniidae.   The main difference between the taeniid egg and that dealt with above is the presence of a greatly thickened embryophore in the former (Fig. 38). The most detailed studies have been carried out on *T. saginata*,[122, 386-7] *T. pisiformis*,[386-7] *T. solium*,[122] *H. taeniaeformis*.[174]

The first stage in the hatching is a darkening of the embryophore, followed by disintegration of the packed keratin blocks comprising the embryophore. It has been assumed by some workers that disintegration is the result of dissolution of a ' cementing ' substance holding these blocks together; but in fact, there is no direct evidence for the existence of such a substance. Ultrastructure studies[248] show only a clear space between the embryophore blocks, a result difficult to explain if a cement substance is present. On the other hand, some workers have described the presence of a highly refractive yellow brown cement substance. Nevertheless, the fact that hatching is brought about by digestive enzymes does suggest that some cementing material is dissolved.

The effect of enzymes on the disintegration of the embryophore varies markedly between species. Pancreatin alone has been reported to bring about hatching in some species, e.g. *T. pisiformis*,[387] *H. taeniaeformis*,[419] *E. granulosus*,[242] although other workers[148] have found pepsin necessary in some cases (Table 33). Eggs of *T. crassiceps* hatch when injected directly into the small intestine,[107] and in *T. solium* some hatching can occur in intestinal juice, although the process is much assisted by pepsin. This raises the question of whether ' auto-infection ' with this species—resulting in cysticercosis—is possible.[122] In contrast, the embryophore of *T. saginata* was found to be unaffected by pancreatin even after 30 hours, but could be disrupted by shaking after 2–3 hours' treatment with pepsin.[386] The conditions under which eggs are stored prior to testing may be an important factor in their ability to hatch, and this may explain the conflicting results of different workers.

Before becoming infective, a released oncosphere must further become ' activated '. ' Activation ' is an interesting phenomenon, the nature of which is not understood. When hatched artificially, an oncosphere first appears still wrapped in its thin oncospheral membrane; the latter is often closely applied to the organism and difficult to see except under phase microscopy. Only a very small number (3% in *T. pisiformis* and *T. saginata*)[386] of free oncospheres show any activity. It is only when bile is added to the hatching medium that an appreciable proportion of embryos show movement. The physiological basis of this onset of activity is not known, but it may be related to the surface active properties of bile. Related to this activity is an increase in the permeability of the oncospheral membrane, which takes place in the presence of bile and pancreatin. This effect may be demonstrated by the use of dyes, such as Nile blue sulphate, neutral red, methylene blue, alizarin, Janus B green and bromophenol blue + nigrosin, which stain the embryo after, but not before, activation.[174, 386] The fact that the oncospheral membrane stains in Nile blue sulphate, but not in the other stains, points to its being a lipoidal membrane. In view of the variation in composition of bile in different species of vertebrates (p. 36), it is likely that bile may play a part in determining intermediate host specificity by selectively activating some species of embryos and not others. Artificial digestive solutions developed by Silverman[386] have been widely used for the hatching and activation of taeniid eggs. Modified solutions utilised for *T. pisiformis*,[148] which have given up to 95% activation, are given in Table 33.

TABLE 33

Artificial gastric and intestinal solutions utilised for hatching the eggs of T. pisi-
formis ; up to 95% *activation may be obtained.   Treatment in roller tubes*
(Data from Heath[148])

Solution A.   *Gastric solution*

0·2% pepsin (3 × cryst. : 1 : 6,000) ⎱ in Hank's saline ... 1 hr.
1·0% HCl   ⎰

Solution B.   *Intestinal solution*

0·5% pancreatin (V) ⎱
1·0% NaHCO₃   ⎰ in dist. H₂O ...   ... 30 mins.
5·0% rabbit bile   ⎰

Even when treated in a similar way, eggs from a particular proglottid of a particular species do not always hatch in a uniform manner. Thus, only 5% eggs of *Hydatigera taeniaeformis*[174] hatched after 1 hour's treatment, 50% after 2 hours and 83% after 3 hours. This variable rate of hatchability may have some advantage in increasing the dissemination of eggs.

Metabolism

No doubt, it is the technical difficulties involved, that have caused the metabolism of cestode eggs to remain almost unstudied. Since cyclophyllidean eggs develop within a proglottid while still within the host, direct examination of the metabolism of development is virtually impossible. Pseudophyllidean eggs, which develop in water, are more suitable for study. Respiration appears to have been studied only in the eggs of *D. latum*.[108, 132] Oxygen consumption is fairly uniform during the first four days of embryonation (at 25°C) and then rises sharply during the 5th and 6th day (Fig. 45). This pattern is comparable to that found in other invertebrate embryos, and presumably reflects the higher synthetic demands of the final stages of morphogenesis of the coracidium. Respiration is unaffected by absence of light, but is completely inhibited by M/1000 KCN.[108]

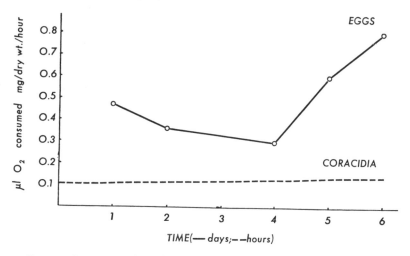

FIG. 45. O_2 consumption of eggs of *Diphyllobothrium latum* at 25°C., 760 mm. Hg, during embryonation. (After Grabiec, Guttowa & Michajlow, 1964.)

In contrast with the egg, the respiration of the hatched coracidia of *D. latum* and that of *Triaenophorus nodulosus* are virtually anaerobic, and only a slight consumption of oxygen can be detected.[132] Poly-saccharides and phospholipids have been detected in the ciliated envelopes (embryophores) of the coracidia of both these species; these become visibly reduced in quantity during the life of the coracidia[131] and presumably represent energy reserves for the larva. Although the cilia on a coracidium beat actively, the contained onco-sphere remains motionless and presumably becomes activated on ingestion by the intermediate host. On hatching, coracidia of both *D. latum* and *T. nodulus* have been found to show some weak orientation towards the anode in an electric field.[131]

In the cyclophyllid egg, glycogen is present during all the stages of embryogenesis;[350-1] the pathways of its metabolism have not been investigated.

8: Developmental Biology of Larvae

General Account

Problems of special physiological interest in larval development include those relating to (a) penetration of the intermediate host gut, (b) migration to the site of development within that host, and (c) resistance to the defence mechanisms of the host. Questions of interest, which arise later in metacestode* development, are those concerned with infection of the second intermediate host (where one occurs) and infection of, and establishment within, the definitive host. Superimposed on these are problems associated with the ecological relationships between the definitive and intermediate host(s)—relationships which often have clear physiological implications. For example, if the first intermediate host of a pseudophyllid is a fresh water copepod, it can normally be assumed that (a) the coracidium will be adapted to fresh water, (b) the second intermediate host will be a freshwater organism (normally a fish) and (c) the definitive host will be a ' waterassociating ' organism (i.e. a fish or a bird).

Most of the detailed studies on the physiology of larvae have been carried out on pseudophyllids; comparatively little is known of the developmental physiology of the Cyclophyllidea, and virtually nothing about the remaining groups. This is understandable, since coracidia are free-swimming and the procercoids frequently develop in sites where continuous observation is not difficult, e.g. the haemocoele of a copepod. Moreover, larval stages of many pseudophyllids may be cultured for long periods *in vitro* (Chapter 10). In contrast, cyclophyllid oncospheres are generally difficult to observe *in situ*.

---

* The term ' metacestode ' is a convenient one to indicate the stage or succession of stages of the tapeworm life cycle that is passed within an intermediate host.[471]

Invasion of the First Intermediate Host

Pseudophyllidea

A series of interesting studies on the invasion of copepods has been carried out.[137, 138, 203]   In particular, an attempt has been made to draw up categories of resistance to infection and to define the barriers to infection. Useful practical techniques for embryonation and hatching of pseudophyllidean eggs and infection of copepods by coracidia have been worked out in considerable detail by Mueller.[253, 254] Coracidia appear to swim in random directions, like gas molecules, spiralling slightly around the central direction of motion. Their specific gravity approaches $1 \cdot 0$ and they are not thrown down by forces in the region of 22 000 g.[253] Copepods do not appear to pursue coracidia actively, even when close to them; nor does visual recognition appear to be involved. Apparently, a coracidium must actively ' collide ' with a copepod in order to be detected as food and eaten.[254]

When a coracidium is ingested by a copepod, three degrees of resistance have been recognised[203] (a) Infection takes place readily and the parasite develops normally; (b) infection occurs, but not readily, and development within the haemocoele is inhibited; (c) only a very low degree of infection occurs, and the development of those larvae which reach the haemocoele is almost completely inhibited. These degrees of resistance have been called *systema obligatorium*, *systema accidentale*, and *systema spurium*,[203] terms which are useful for the purposes of discussion, but which throw no light on the underlying basis for the resistance.

When a coracidium is ingested, it must overcome a number of ' barriers ' before it can reach the haemocoele and develop there. These have been termed ' selective ' barriers, in the sense that their operation is responsible, in part at least, for selecting the particular species of coracidia which can develop in a particular host. These may thus play a part in determining host-specificity. Within a copepod, the major barriers appear to be the digestive juices, the nature of the alimentary canal and the nature of the body cavity contents. In the case of cyclophyllidean eggs, the digestive juices of vertebrate hosts play a part in hatching and hence could act as selective agents. Similarly. surface-active substances, such as bile, are concerned in hatching, besides acting as powerful selective agents for the establishment of adult worms (p. 147). Unfortunately, very little is known about the presence or composition of surface-active agents in invertebrates; it would be especially interesting to know if such substances exist in copepods.

The thickness of the gut wall is probably the major barrier to coracidium penetration, and although there is no quantitative evidence on this point, in some copepods there appears to be a marked increase of resistance to infection with age.[419] Thus, in *Schistocephalus solidus*, the copepodid stages of *Cyclops* are easily infected, whereas the adults are almost entirely resistant. In the case of *Spirometra mansonoides*, a wide variation in infectivity has been reported, and factors such as whether coracidia are from early or late hatches appear to be involved.[254] Presumably, coracidia which have been swimming for prolonged periods before ingestion by a copepod, may be so low in energy reserves that they are unable to penetrate the gut wall. That energy reserves are important is borne out by the fact that, at 18–20°C, a high degree of infectivity is maintained for 36–48 hours but at lower temperatures (10–15°C) ability to infect lasts 2–4 days.[138]

Following ingestion by a copepod, a coracidium rapidly becomes liberated from the ciliated envelope (embryophore)—presumably by the action of digestive enzymes.[137] A freed oncosphere then rapidly penetrates the gut wall. This process appears to be aided by the hook movements, for, unlike the hexacanth embryo of many cyclophyllids, pseudophyllid coracidia lack 'penetration glands' (p. 129), so that penetration of the copepod gut may be largely mechanical.

Cyclophyllidea

Although descriptive accounts of the infection of the intermediate host by hatched cyclophyllid oncospheres have been given, little appears to be known of the physiology of the process. The few accounts of gut penetration given have been confined to those species which utilise arthropod (especially insect) intermediate hosts, and in which the processes of penetration can be followed, e.g. *Dipylidium caninum*[63] and *Oochoristica vacuolata*.[157]

In addition to the mechanical action of the hooks, histolytic enzymes are almost certainly involved, because well-defined ' penetration '[325] or ' epidermal ' glands (Figs. 46, 47) have been described in numerous species: *Raillietina cesticillus*,[325] *R. echinobothrida* and *R. kashiwarensis*,[360] *Choanotaenia infundibulum, Moniezia expansa, Hymenolepis* spp.,[269, 272, 325] *Mesocestoides corti*,[419] *Oochoristica symmetrica*,[270] *O. vacuolata*,[157] *O. ratti*,[327] *O. deserti*,[243] *Davainea proglottina*,[98] *Atriotaenia procyonis*,[111] *Taenia pisiformis*,[386] *T. saginata*,[387] and *Dilepis undula*.[271]

The chemical contents of the glands have not been determined, although it is known[360, 361, 390] that they are PAS-positive. The glands can also be stained by vital dyes and are visible by means of phase contrast microscopy. Oncosphere cytology is best studied in aceto-orcein preparations.[274]

In the mouse intestine, oncospheres have been shown to lyse the cement substances between the cells and also to possess cytolytic properties, which assist in penetration.[390]   A similar effect has been demonstrated in the penetration of the rabbit intestine by *Taenia* oncospheres; in this case the cells themselves are actually lysed.[148]

That the gland secretions are, in fact, concerned in penetration, is

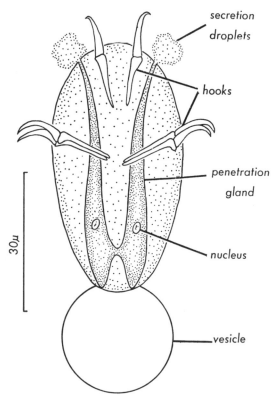

FIG. 46. An activated hexacanth larva of *Raillietina cesti-cillus* showing secretion from penetration glands. (Based on Reid, 1948.)

supported by the observation that in *R. cesticillus* they failed to give a PAS reaction after penetration of the gut of the intermediate beetle host.[361]   Other workers, however, have not confirmed this result.[148] Some secretion also occurs during the hatching of the egg and the secretion may assist in the perforation of the larval membranes.[148, 361] Release of parasite secretions during penetration has some immuno-logical significance; for such materials undoubtedly act as exogenous antigens (p. 207). As might be expected in a rapid protein-synthesising system, the oncosphere is rich in RNA.[350]

In addition to the normal method of egg infection *per os*, several artificial methods of infection of vertebrate hosts have been successful. Cattle have been infected with cysticerci by subcutaneous or intra-muscular injections of hatched oncospheres of *T. saginata*.[109] Rather surprisingly, intravenous or epidural injections—which might have been expected more closely to approximate the natural infection route—

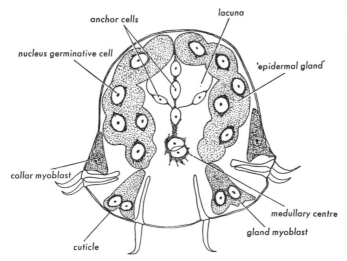

Fig. 47. An oncosphere of *Hymenolepis diminuta*, showing cytology. (After Ogren, 1962.)

failed to give positive results.   It is also well known, that *Echinococcus* can be transmitted to the intermediate host by intraperitoneal injections of protoscoleces.[268]

Growth and Differentiation of Metacestodes

Pseudophyllidea

Procercoid. Studies on growth and differentiation of larvae within this group have been confined to a few genera, especially *Schistocephalus*, *Ligula*, *Diphyllobothrium* and *Spirometra*.   In both the procercoid and plerocercoid of pseudophyllids there is a tendency towards progenesis (advanced development of genitalia in a larva without maturation), and neoteny (maturation of gonads in a larva).   The full range of larval development normally involves the successive stages: oncosphere, procercoid, plerocercoid, and adult. However, in the most advanced neotenic form, *Archigetes*, the procercoid stage may reach maturity in the body cavity of its first intermediate host (a tubificid oligochaete). although maturation may also occur in a fish.[189] In *Bothriocephalus claviceps*[182] the procercoid develops in a copepod and reaches maturity directly in the gut of *Anguilla anguilla*, i.e. without a plerocercoid stage

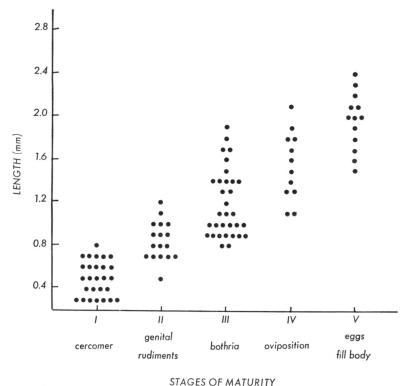

FIG. 48. *Archigetes limnodrili*—length at each stage of maturity; the measurements do not include the cercomer. (After Kennedy, 1965.)

in a second intermediate host being required in the life cycle. In the fully extended life cycle, as exemplified by *D. latum*, the plerocercoid develops in fish viscera and the adult usually in the gut of warm-blooded vertebrates.

Apparently nothing is known about the factors controlling the development of somatic and germinal tissues of these larva. The common occurrence of neoteny in the group suggests that these growth processes may operate independently of each other; they may prove to be much more loosely linked than would be normally expected in a metazoan organism.

The growth rate of procercoids in copepods has been examined for only a few species, e.g. *D. latum*[137, 138] and *S. solidus*[69] The growth rate of *Archigetes limnodrili* in freshwater oligochaetes has also been studied (Fig. 48).[189] Growth of the procercoids of *S. solidus* follows a smooth curve and shows no unusual pattern (Fig. 49). The stage at which a procercoid becomes infective is marked by the appearance of the cercomer, a tail-like appendage containing the oncospheral hooks

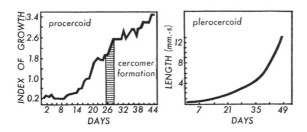

Fig. 49. Growth of the procercoid and plerocercoid of *Schistocephalus solidus*. (Adapted from Clarke, 1954.)

(Fig. 50), the significance of which is not understood. The rate of growth in the copepod host is more or less inversely proportional to the degree of infection[138]—presumably a nutritional phenomenon. In unfavourable copepod hosts, inhibition of growth of *D. latum* is almost complete, and the undeveloped coracidia become absorbed. The nature of this process is not understood, but it may be related to 'immune' phenomena (e.g. phagocytosis). Even well-developed procercoids may be absorbed and the disintegration of the procercoids of *Ligula colymbi*, after they had reached an advanced state of development in copepods, has been reported.[419]

Procercoids are typically provided with what appears to be a well-developed gland (Fig. 50), which opens by anterior ducts. Neither the structure of this gland nor the nature of its secretion has been examined. It may release a histolytic secretion—perhaps a collagenase, which could assist in penetration, as in trematode cercariae.[422]

Plerocercoid. It has been stressed (p. 131) that pseudophyllid larvae in general, show a tendency towards progenesis and neoteny. This is evidenced by an examination of the life cycles of *Diphyllobothrium*, *Ligula*, *Digramma*, *Schistocephalus*, *Amphilina*, *Caryophyllaeus*, *Biacetabulum* and *Archigetes*,[95] and has apparently resulted in evolution in the direction of decreasing the number of hosts and of transferring sexual development to the larval phases.

In the genus *Diphyllobothrium*, the plerocercoid is morphologically undifferentiated, genital anlagen are almost entirely absent, and most species require at least seven days to reach maturity in a warm-blooded host.[419]   In contrast, the plerocercoids of *Ligula*, *Schistocephalus*, and *Digramma* are progenetic and possess sufficient food reserves, so that a relatively simple stimulus is all that is required to induce rapid maturation.   That rise in temperature provides this stimulus has been

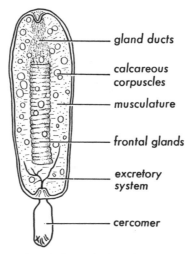

— gland ducts

— calcareous corpuscles

— musculature

— frontal glands

— excretory system

— cercomer

FIG. 50. A typical pseudophyllidean procercoid. (From Smyth, 1962b; based on Kuhlow 1963.)

unequivocally demonstrated in *Ligula* and *Schistocephalus*, by maturing these species *in vitro* (p. 169) at 40°C.[14, 405, 407, 415]   A temperature stimulus similarly induces maturation in *Digramma interrupta*; and by raising the aquarium temperature, maturation of the plerocercoid, whilst still within its intermediate fish host, has been achieved.[95]

As might be expected, the growth rate of the plerocercoids in fish markedly increases with rise in temperature.   Thus, plerocercoids of *Diphyllobothrium sebago*, in trout in a water temperature of 1°C (Dec.–March), grew to only 1–2 mm after 113 days; but after an additional 61 days (April–May), during which time the temperature rose to 10°C, larvae grew to 12–15 mm.[241]

Certain species (e.g. *Proteocephalus filicollis*), which mature in freshwater fish in temperate climates, go through an annual cycle of infection and maturation; and in them, too, maturation appears to be associated with a seasonal rise in environmental temperature.[164]

At the lower end of the temperature scale, it has been shown that plerocercoids are remarkably resistant to low temperatures.   Plerocercoids of *D. latum* in a 70 gm perch can survive for 20 days at 0°C, but only for much shorter periods at lower temperatures: 72 hrs. at −5°C, 8 hrs at −15°C, and 2 hrs. at −40°C.[419]   At temperatures below −8°C, death appears to be due to ice formation.[481]

There have been few detailed studies on the biochemistry of growth of plerocercoids.   The water and glycogen content of the plerocercoid of *Schistocephalus* during growth have been studied,[233] and it has been shown that (i) between 5 and 15 mg fresh weight (1–3 mg dry weight), the percentage water content changes little, (ii) between 15 and 100 mg fresh weight (3–30 mg dry weight) the % dry weight rises rapidly, the water content falling from over 80% to 68-69%, (iii) over 100 mg fresh weight, the dry weight again becomes stable.   The glycogen content closely mimics the change in water content, the most characteristic feature being a phase between 15 and 100 mg fresh weight— when the percentage glycogen increases rapidly—at an exponential rate. This change may be associated with the fact that at about 15 mg (fresh weight) the plerocercoids first develop distinct genital primordia and become capable of maturation if subjected to the appropriate temperature rise.[170]

From *in vitro* studies with *Schistocephalus*, it has been found that 'small' plerocercoids were metabolically much more active than 'larger', i.e. old, plerocercoids; thus, the *specific* growth rate (i.e. that for any particular-sized larva) of a 4 mg (dry weight) worm was shown to be 8–10 times that of a 40 mg worm.[232]   The specific growth rate of a *Schistocephalus* plerocercoid is given by the equation:

$$g = aw^b$$

where g = specific growth rate; w = mean weight of plerocercoid; a and b constants.

The maximal growth rate of *Schistocephalus* plerocercoids occurs between 23 and 27°C,[394] and the 'larval' enzyme systems probably operate up to 30°C.   Above this temperature, the metabolism is believed to switch to the 'adult' system, which can result in growth to maturity.[92, 394]

The cell population kinetics of the plerocercoids of *Diphyllobothrium osmeri* and *D. latum*, with particular reference to the effect of temperature, has been examined.[480]   In a marathon study, Wikgren[480] counted the number of cells in a single plerocercoid of *D. osmeri* and by colchicine treatment determined the percentage of mitoses (Table 34). Mitosis did not occur in the subcuticular region and, in all, some 42% of the cells were differentiated and were mitotically inactive; differentiated cells include subcuticular cells, flame cells and calcareous corpuscle cells.

TABLE 34

The composition of the cell population of plerocercoids of Diphyllobothrium osmeri. *The number of cells in a quarter of a section of each of* 10 *plerocercoids was counted. The percentages of flame cells and cells associated with the calcareous corpuscles were determined from separate sections. The plerocercoids were treated for five hours with colchicine*
(Data from Wikgren[480])

	Sub-cuticle	Outer paren-chyma	Muscle layer	Inner paren-chyma
Total no. of cells	2,586	2,088	972	1,271
Percentage of flame cells	0	6·5	0	0
Percentage of calcareous corpuscle cells	0	6·6	0	5·2
Total no. of mitotically inactive cells	2,586	274	0	66
No. of parenchymal cells	0	1,814	972	1,205
No. of mitoses	0	52	129	92
Percentage of mitoses	0	2·9	13·3	7·6

In view of the marked influence of temperature on development, it is not surprising to find that the rate of entry of cells into mitosis is very sensitive to temperature, varying from 0·1 cell/100 cells/hr at 10°C to 1·9 cell/100 cells/hr. at 38°C. The temperature response of the main parameters of mitosis almost exactly follows the pattern observed in other biological material (Table 35). The doubling time of the whole cell population was estimated to be 54 hrs. at 38°C, and 960 hours at 10°C.[480]

TABLE 35

The duration of mitosis and its various stages at four temperatures in Diphyllobothrium osmeri. *The duration of the stages was obtained by direct apportioning of the duration of mitosis according to the frequences : prophases* 14 *per cent, metaphases* 72 *per cent and anaphases* 14 *per cent.*
(Data from Wikgren[480])

		Duration (minutes) of :		
Temperature	Complete mitosis	Prophase (late)	Metaphase	Anaphase
10	223	31	161	31
20	96	13	70	13
30	29	4	21	4
38–39	13	2	9	2

Cyclophyllidea

(i) *Larvae with an invertebrate intermediate host*

Most of the studies on growth rate and development have been carried out on *H. nana* and *H. diminuta*.[467] As can be expected, temperature is one of the major factors affecting the rate of development in the intermediate host. The cysticercoids of *H. diminuta* develop in 5 days at 37°C, but require 65 days at 15°C[468]. Temperatures higher than 37°C appear to inhibit cysticercoid development and induce abnormalities.[460-2] Excessively heavy infections in arthropod hosts can also induce abnormal development. Thus, in copepods infected with more than 7–10 larvae of *Drepanidotaenia lanceolata*, the normal rate of development was disturbed.[202] In the haemocoele, competition for available nutrients could clearly occur, and in the case of *Diorchis ransomi* in ostracods the cyst size has been shown to be inversely proportional to the number of contained larvae.[346]

(ii) *Larvae with a vertebrate intermediate host*

(a) *Growth Rate.* Not many studies on the growth rate of this group of larvae have been made and these appear to have been confined to the Taeniidae. The oncosphere of *Hydatigera taeniaeformis* weighs about 1 millimicrogram when first established in a mouse liver[177] but grows to 1 mg after 40 days, i.e. an increase in weight by a factor of 10^6. After this, the rate of growth (defined as the time taken to double its weight) decreases sharply and, in the case of light infections, growth virtually stops by 22 weeks. After this period there is continued inhibition of growth, possibly due to the influence of a host tissue reaction. In the same species, it was shown that the nitrogen content of the strobilocercus fell from above 6% at 42 days (Fig. 51) to less than 4·5% at 67 days, remaining constant after this age at 4·25%+0·25.[168] As this is approximately the time at which a larva becomes infective, it is possible that a relationship, at present inexplicable, exists between the nitrogen level and infectivity.

Although the majority of cestode species form only one larva from one oncosphere, a number of species undergo asexual budding. This is a phenomenon of some theoretical interest, for it touches on fundamental problems of growth and differentiation. Asexual budding appears to be confined to the *Diphyllobothriidae, Hymenolepididae* and *Taeniidae.* The best known species is probably *Echinococcus granulosus* which forms the well known ' hydatid ' cyst and provides unusually interesting material for experimental work. This is related to the fact that a cyst—which itself is formed from a single oncosphere—gives rise by polyembryony (p. 5) to a large number of protoscoleces. Each protoscolex is thus part of a clone, and hence the whole population has the same genetic constitution—an unusual situation for a metazoan organism. It is thus possible to carry out experiments with many thousands of organisms each with an identical genotype.

(b)   *Nutrition.* The study of the nutrition of a larva *in situ*, within a vertebrate intermediate host, clearly raises difficult technical problems and apparently no direct studies have been made. From the physiological point of view, questions of especial interest which arise are

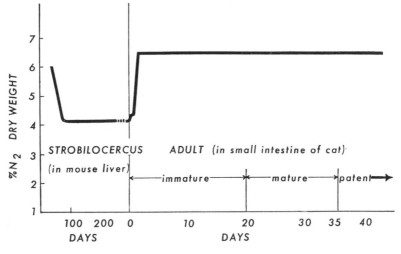

FIG. 51. Variation in nitrogen level in larval and adult *Hydatigera taeniaeformis* with age. The level drops until about the time the strobilocercus becomes infective (63-65 days) when it steadies about 4·25%. (Adapted from Hopkins & Hutchinson, 1958.)

(*a*) Does a larva develop at different rates in different tissue sites? (*b*) What is the nature of the host-parasite interface in such sites? (*c*) What mechanisms of membrane transport are utilised for the transference of nutrients into the growing larva? Little information is available concerning these questions. Thus, it has been shown that in *Taenia crassiceps* the growth rate differs markedly in different sites. This species is a useful laboratory model, since it can be maintained in mice by serial subinoculation of cysticerci;[107] Fig. 52 shows the growth of larval *T. crassiceps* by budding (*a*) in subcutaneous tissue, (*b*) in the pleural cavity and (*c*) in the abdominal cavity. In the subcutaneous focus, at about 40 days, retardation of growth occurs and the growth rate drops until about 150 days, whereafter it becomes steady. In contrast, in the abdominal cavity, growth commences slowly and increases until retardation occurs, this time at 300 days. In the pleural cavity growth is much more limited, but again retardation finally sets in. The retardation observed in all these sites may be due, in part at least, to a tissue reaction.

Since metacestodes occur primarily in tissue sites, it is clear that their nutritional and immunological (p. 190) problems are somewhat analagous to those of mammalian embryos. This analogy has been

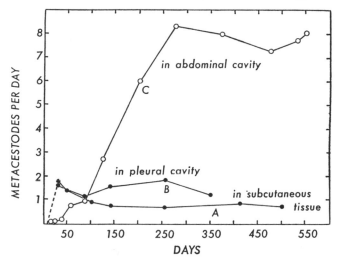

FIG. 52. Rate of reproduction of metacestodes of *Taenia crassiceps* in three different foci in the mouse. (After Freeman, 1962.)

emphasised by Šlais,[400-402] who has drawn attention (Fig. 53) to the following points:

(*a*) The early development of the cestode and the mammalian embryo is analogous.

(*b*) The later development, in which the separation of the embryo from the trophoblast—due to the formation of the umbilical cord—shows a close resemblance to the developmental situation in a cysticercus.

(*c*) The foetal membranes enclose and protect the mammalian embryo; in an analogous manner, the cysticercus bladder folds over and encloses the scolex region.

(*d*) Since the cysticercus bladder wall is the only region in contact with host tissue, it must be assumed that it serves as a nutritional organ analogous with the trophoblast of the mammalian embryo.

This view is based almost entirely on morphological and theoretical considerations, and it will be interesting to see how closely the physiology of the bladder follows that of the placenta.   Unfortunately, almost nothing is known of the transport of metabolites into the cysticercus bladder and, in particular, whether active transport and pinocytosis is involved.   The few ultrastructure studies carried out have not thrown much light on these problems.   In the hydatid cyst of *E. granulosus*, the region of the parasite which makes contact with the host tissue is the ' germinal ' membrane and this is drawn out into villus-like processes

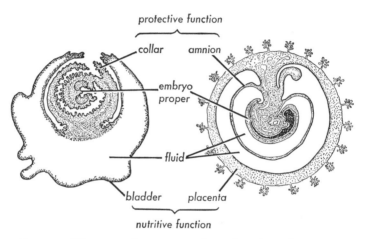

FIG. 53. Diagrammatic representation of analogy between a cysticercus and a mammalian embryo.   (After Šlais, 1966b.)

(Plate IV, Fig. B.) which extend into the laminated layer of the cyst;[251] such processes could be compared with the villi of a placenta.   These processes are surrounded by a membrane and a clear space and some-what resemble the microtriches of the protoscolex (p. 182).   The basal portion contains numerous vacuole-like spaces resembling the vesicles in the tegument of adult cestodes.   No evidence for pinocytosis has been observed.

The ultrastructure of the bladder wall of *Multiceps serialis* has also been examined.[293]   Rather surprisingly, the cyst was found to have a structure almost identical with that of the adult cestode tegument, consisting of long narrow microtriches, extending from a highly vacuo-lated distal cytoplasm.   Again, there was no evidence of pinocytosis.

It is clear from these few studies that little is known regarding the physiology or ultrastructure of the host-parasite interface in larval forms and this is an area in which there appears to be much scope for further work.

Metabolism

The metabolism of the better known and larger larval forms such, as those of *E. granulosus*, *H. taeniaeformis* and *S. solidus*, has already been discussed with the adult metabolism (p. 41) and, in general, only special problems related to the Pseudophyllidea will be mentioned here.

In the pseudophyllids, the plerocercoids are characterised by being rich in glycogen reserves, which may reach 50% dry weight in the case of the progenetic plerocercoids of *Ligula intestinalis* and *S. solidus* (Table 9). These levels of glycogen are exceptionally high, and the availability of such food reserves means that rapid maturation in the definitive host is possible without the absorption of exogenous carbohydrate. Both these species can be matured *in vitro* even in non-nutrient media, provided the usual physico-chemical conditions are controlled (Chapter 10). During *in vitro* maturation, the glycogen level of *Schistocephalus* plerocercoids falls rapidly, more being consumed under anaerobic than aerobic conditions.[163]

Few studies on the nitrogen metabolism have been made. In the plerocercoid of *Diphyllobothrium*[13] the protein composition remains nearly constant throughout growth from 3 to 30 mg (fresh weight), but rises rapidly during maturation in the final host. The level in worms which migrate into the anterior two-thirds of the gut is lower than those remaining in the posterior one-third (Fig. 16). This apparent anomaly is probably related to a *relative* increase in glycogen in the anteriorly situated worms.

Pseudophyllid plerocercoids have been reported as inducing some interesting physiological, as well as pathological, effects on their hosts.[485] For example, the plerocercoids of *Ligula intestinalis* induce parasitic castration in the fish, *Leuciscus rutilus*—a condition which is associated with a reduction of the basophil cells in the middle glandular region of the pituitary.[15, 197] This is accompanied by a reduction of the level of gonadotrophic hormones secreted.[201] Parasitic castration is not induced by the plerocercoids of *Schistocephalus* in the fish *Gasterosteus aculeatus*.[171, 197] Although oocyte maturation is delayed, unlike *Ligula*, this effect does not appear to be due to suppression of pituitary activity since the pituitary appears to be cytologically normal.[15] Other pathological effects induced by plerocercoids of *Schistocephalus* include a fall in blood cell volume, liver glycogen and liver weight in infected fish. Some degree of parasitic castration is also induced in earthworms by cysts of *Paricterotaenia paradoxa*.[376] The breeding behaviour of fish infected with *Ligula* or *Schistocephalus* is also affected.[15, 277]

Perhaps the most remarkable metabolic effect associated with infection of plerocercoids has been described for *Spirometra mansonoides*.[259-262] Mueller[259] made the unexpected observation that when spargana (plerocercoids) of this species were injected subcutaneously into young mice, the host gained weight at a rate which could not be accounted for by the weight of the parasites or the associated tissue reaction. The difference in weight increase between these mice and the control mice could easily be judged by the eye (Plate III). An even greater weight increase was found in deer mice (*Peromyscus*) and hamsters.[260] A similar stimulating effect has also been described for an oriental species, *Sparganum ranarum*.[260]

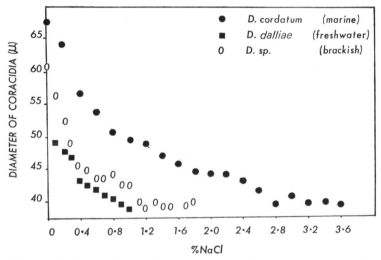

FIG. 54. Influence of osmotic pressure on the diameter of the coracidia of *Diphyllobothrium* spp. (After Hilliard, 1960.)

Since plerocercoids contain large quantities of carbohydrate reserves, these results suggested that hormones controlling these reserves were leaking into the host system.[262] In support of this view, it has been found that epididymal adipose tissue from infected mice stimulated glucose oxidation, utilisation of glucose for lipogenesis and cell penetration of D-galactose. These are well-known effects elicited by the hormone insulin; which suggests that *Spirometra* releases an insulin-like substance into the host.[1-412] Mice infected with *Spirometra* also had a postabsorptive hyperglycaemia, depressed levels of serum alkaline phosphatase and reduced amounts of serum total protein.[354]

Although the plerocercoid stages of the Diphyllobothridae and the

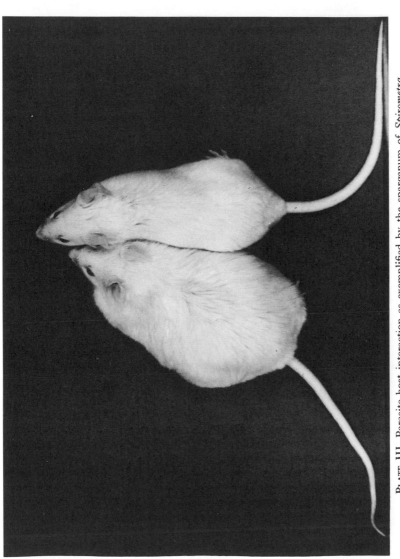

PLATE III. Parasite-host interaction as exemplified by the sparganum of *Spirometra mansonoides*. The parasite releases an insulin-like substance which stimulates glucose oxidation in the host. *Left*: experimental mouse infected (subcutaneously) with 8 spargana for 64 days. *Right*: uninfected control. (After Mueller, 1963.)

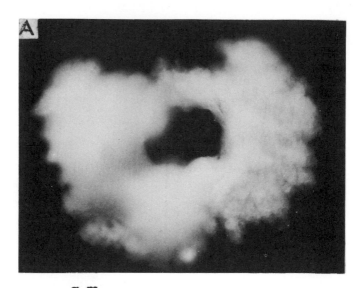

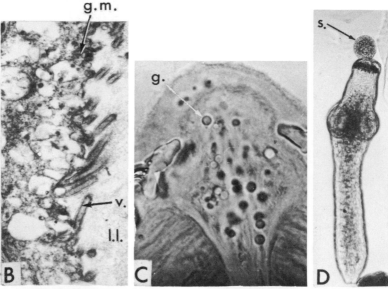

Plate IV. A. Precipitate formed around scolex of sparganum of *Spirometra mansonoides in vitro* culture; probably a reaction of scolex gland secretion with protein in medium. (After Mueller, 1961b.) B. Electron micrograph of hydatid cyst wall showing villus-like processes (v.) projecting from germinal membrane (g.m.) into laminated layer (l.l.). (After Morseth, 1967a.) C. Section of *Echinococcus granulosus* showing globules of secretion (g.) in cells of rostellar gland. (After Smyth, 1964a.) D. Precipitates formed at the rostellar tip of *Echinococcus granulosus* during *in vitro* culture; probably a reaction of rostellar gland secretion with ' non-specific antibody ' in culture medium. (Original.)

cysticercus and strobilocercus stages of Taeniidae have been extensively studied, almost nothing is known of the physiology of the coracidium, the procercoid and the cysticercoid stages. This position is undoubtedly related to technical difficulties associated with size and handling. The few observations made on the coracidium have shown—rather unexpectedly—that its respiration is essentially anaerobic (Fig. 45). Coracidia of different species appear to have a tissue osmotic pressure related to the biotope of the definitive host.[158] The coracidium of *Diphyllobothrium cordatum*, for example, swells rapidly in distilled water (Fig. 54) but at sea water levels (2·8% NaCl) larvae retained their minimum diameter. In contrast, the coracidium of *D. dalliae* has an osmotic pressure equivalent to about 1% NaCl (Fig. 54) and presumably could be classified as a freshwater species. Another undefined species of *Diphyllobothrium* lies between these two extremes and can be considered a brackish-water species.

The metabolism of the procercoid *in vivo* is virtually unknown. In the copepod, *Eudiaptomus gracilis*, infected with procercoids of *Triaenophorus nodulosus*, it has been shown that the free amino acids in the general pool of amino acids in the haemolymph fell from 35·4% in normal copepods to 13% in infected specimens. The amino acids which decreased were lysine, aspartic acid, tyrosine, tryptophane and phenylalanine, suggesting that these amino acids are essential for growth and development for this species of cestode.[139]

9: Development Within Definitive Host

Mechanism of Invasion

With the exception of a few neotenic forms (e.g. *Archigetes*), in which infection of the definitive host takes place directly via the egg, a host normally becomes infected by ingesting an intermediate host containing a metacestode. Metacestodes may occur in the intermediate host in any of the four states: (*i*) free, (*ii*) encysted, (*iii*) encapsulated, (*iv*) both encysted and encapsulated. The term *encysted* is used when the cyst is produced by the parasite; *encapsulated* when it is produced by the host. In the latter case, the cyst may sometimes consist of two layers, the outer of which is derived from the host and the inner from the larva. In some larvae (e.g. *Echinococcus*) the borderline between host and parasite tissue is difficult to detect.

The metacestode scolex is normally invaginated or withdrawn— a measure which presumably protects the scolex until it is stimulated to evaginate in the appropriate region of the host gut. To become established in the gut, therefore, a larva must (*a*) free itself of its surrounding membranes (i.e. excyst), (*b*) evaginate its scolex, (*c*) become ' activated ', (*d*) become attached to the intestinal mucosa.

Excystment and Evagination

General Account

Although excystment and evagination are theoretically separate processes, in many cases the second follows so closely after the first that they cannot readily be distinguished. In some species, a particular enzyme may be required to digest the cystic membrane completely before the larva escapes; in others, the same enzyme may so activate the larva that it breaks out of its enveloping membranes before they are fully digested. Requirements for excystment and evagination in particular species are summarised in Table 36. For these results to be meaningful, the precise experimental conditions under which they were obtained must be known.   In a few cases, e.g. *Echinococcus*,[423] *Hydatigera*,[339] pepsin alone is sufficient to cause excystment.   In most cases, however, trypsin and/or pancreatin in the presence of bile is necessary for excystment and evagination.   Pepsin normally has an enhancing effect, but may not be necessary for some species (Table 36).

TABLE 36

Requirements for excystment and evagination of some cyclophyllidean metacestodes; for these results to be of value the duration of treatment and the physico-chemical conditions of the medium must be taken into account

$+$ = essential ; $-$ = non essential ;   . = no information ;   E = enhance effect.

Species	Pepsin	Trypsin	Lipase	Pancre-atin	Bile Salt	Reference
Hydatigera taeniaeformis	$+$	$-$	.	$-$	$-$	339
Oochoristica symmetrica	$-$	$-$	.	.	$+$	339
Hymenolepis diminuta	E	$+$	.	.	$+$	339
Hymenolepis citelli	E	$+$	.	.	$+$	339
Hymenolepis nana	E	$+$	.	.	$+$	339
Taenia solium	$+$	$-$?	.	.	$+$	339
Taenia pisiformis	$-$	$-$	.	.	$+$	353a
Raillietina kashiwarensis	$-$	$+$	$-$	$+$	$-$	357
Raillietina cesticillus	$-$	$-$	.	.	$+$	301
Paricterotaenia paradoxa	$+$	.	.	$+$	$-$	377
*Echinococcus granulosus**	$+^a/E^b$	$+^b$	.	$+^b$	$+$	^{b}353, ^{a}423

* See pp. 145–6

A hydatid cyst of *E. granulosus*, containing brood capsules with proto-scoleces, is large enough to be torn open (= excysted?) by the teeth of the dog. *In vitro*, however, pepsin is needed to free a high proportion of the protoscoleces from the brood capsule membranes, 10 mins treatment with 0·025% crystalline pepsin at pH 2·0 being sufficient to digest the membranes.[423]   Although evagination of the protoscoleces is greatly accelerated by bile (see below) almost the same degree of evagination (but not necessarily activation) is reached *without* this treatment, but the *rate* of evagination is slower (Fig. 55).[423] The physico-chemical conditions pH, E_h, pO_2, pCO_2, under which evagination takes place do not appear, as such, to have been examined in detail. Protoscoleces of *E. granulosus* will not evaginate under anaerobic conditions—but do so at a 10% O_2 level.[423]   Storage of protoscoleces of *Echinococcus* at 2°C, has also been reported as inhibiting evagination.[353] The pseudophyllidean scolex appears to evaginate more readily than the cyclophyllidean scolex.   Some small species e.g. *Diphyllobothrium* sp., evaginate and even become attached to the wall of a culture tube in bile-less media such as saline or broth, although some of the larger species e.g. *S. mansonoides*, require bile and enzyme treatment.[29]

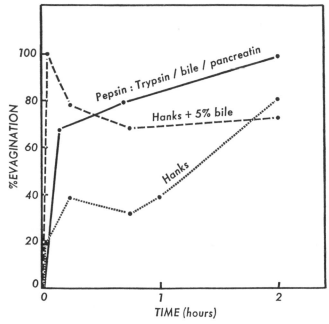

FIG. 55. Evagination of protoscoleces of *Echinococcus granulosus* with and without bile and/or enzyme treatment. (After Smyth, 1967.)

Role of Bile

It has long been known that bile salts can stimulate evagination of the scolex, as well as acting synergistically with digestive enzymes to digest the cyst membranes as shown above. Bile is also known to play a part in the excystment of the metacercarial cysts of trematodes[422] and the oocysts of coccidia.[426] The action of bile on cestode larvae appears to be to stimulate peristaltic movement, but the basis for this phenomenon is not known.

Since a number of artificial surfactants (e.g. Haemo-Sol.) have been shown to stimulate evagination in the cysticerci of *T. pisiformis*, it is likely that surface tension effects play a major part in this process, a tension of about 50–60 dynes/cm² being effective in most cases.[56] In addition, however, chemical effects are almost certainly involved; for some surfactants have inhibitory effects. Also, as shown below, bile, although a surfactant, cannot induce and maintain evagination by itself in most species, and enzymes or other co-factors may be necessary.

Since a wide range of bile acids occurs in vertebrates (Table 8), it may be expected that the composition of bile—along with other factors (p. 25)—may determine whether or not a particular species can develop in a particular host. In other words, bile may represent a biochemical factor determining host specificity. Hence, in a host, the exposed surface of a successful established · parasite must have a molecular configuration not susceptible to attack by the various surface-active agents present in bile. For instance, the cuticle of *Echinococcus* is rapidly lysed by deoxycholic acid, and biles from 'unsuitable' hosts such as hare, rabbit or sheep—which are rich in this acid—rapidly lyse the cuticle. In contrast, biles from 'suitable' carnivore hosts, such as the fox, dog and cat—which are relatively poor in deoxycholic acid— have no such lytic effect.[416] The type of conjugation of the bile acid, i.e. whether linked to taurine or glycine, may also prove to be important.

Bile may act as a ' selection ' agent in two ways, either by a particular type or concentration of bile salt being necessary for evagination, establishment or growth of a particular cestode species, or alternatively bile could act as a toxic or lytic agent in an unfavourable host.

The composition of bile salts is extremely complex[146] and bile salts are unusually difficult to obtain in a pure condition; much of the work done on cestodes utilising bile salts of commercial origin, must therefore, be accepted with reservation.

Establishment in Host Intestine

The actual process of establishment in the host intestine has been examined in only a few instances. Several species have been shown to undergo a forward migration after initial attachment in a more posterior region. Thus, *H. diminuta* first establishes itself about 40 cm posterior to the stomach and then moves forward after 7–10 days of growth.[419] Again, *H. microstoma* first establishes itself in the duodenum and then migrates to the bile duct after four days.[352] Similarly, *D. dendriticum* establishes itself initially in the large intestine of rats, but migrates forwards to the duodenum within twenty-four hours.[12] In contrast, *R. cesticillus* migrates in the opposite direction,[106] originally attaching anterior to the bile duct but moving backwards after three days (Fig. 56).

In some species, which have a wide host spectrum, the position established in the gut, as well as the length of life, varies from host to host. In the case of *Schistocephalus solidus*, which can mature in both avian and mammalian hosts, the best level of establishment was in 1–4 week old ducks ($>50\%$ established) and 2–5 week old chicks (nearly 40% established); establishment was also possible in rats and hamsters.[232] After six hours, this species occupied a specific region of the intestine in different hosts (Fig. 57).

The ability of worms to establish themselves also appears to be determined genetically. When *H. nana* was selfed—by establishing single infections in mice (to insure self fertilisation)—three main effects

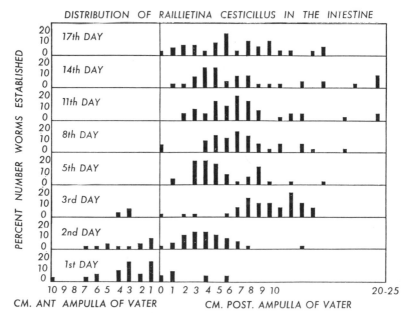

FIG. 56. Distribution of *Raillietina cesticillus* in the fowl intestine after initial infection. (After Foster & Daugherty, 1959.)

were noted: (*a*) marked decrease in infectivity of cysticercoids, (*b*) decrease in infectivity of eggs and (*c*) increase in percentage of abnormal cysticercoids produced.[331] In this experiment, worms in the control rats, each of which had been infected with 6 cysticercoids, also declined in infectivity (Fig. 58). This result suggests that, at this low level of infection, selfing, not cross-fertilisation, takes place.

In *E. granulosus*, where the infective larvae (protoscoleces) are small, at least some establish themselves within the crypts of Lieberkühn during the early stages of infection, but later move out towards the lumen as the scolex, and especially the suckers, grow in size. The majority finally become established with the rostellum pushed into a crypt and the suckers grasping the base of the villi

(Fig. 12).   A small proportion of worms break through into the *lamina propria*.[425]

If a scolex has a rostellum and suckers of a certain size, it is obvious— as dealt with earlier (p. 26)—that this factor could play an important role in determining host-specificity.[483]   The more closely a scolex is

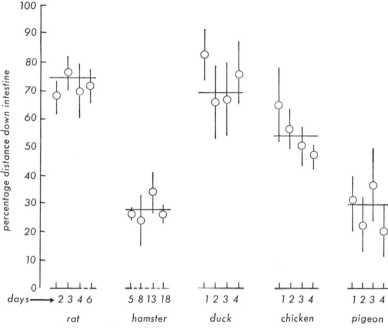

FIG. 57. Position of the pseudophyllidean cestode, *Schistocephalus solidus* when established in different laboratory hosts. (After McCaig & Hopkins, 1963.)

adapted to the morphology of a particular type of mucosa, the narrower the host spectrum is likely to be.   In this respect, the Pseudophyllidea may prove to be generally less host-specific than the Cyclophyllidea, although it is difficult to generalise.   Thus *D. dendriticum*, which develops normally in the gulls *Larus canus*, *L. argentatus* and *L. ridibundus*, can also develop in rats.[417]   However, although many species of Cyclophyllidea, e.g. *Taenia solium*, are confined to one host, others—such as *H. nana*—have a wide host range.[369]   Thus, *H. nana* can develop in mice, hamsters and grey squirrels,[367] although the growth rate and pattern of development differs in each host (Fig. 59). Many factors are clearly likely to be involved in determining host specificity.

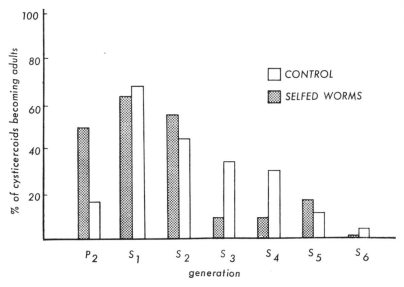

Fig. 58. Loss of viability in *Hymenolepis nana*, related to selfing through six generations; measured as percentage of cysticercoids becoming adults. P_2, progeny of P_1 generation; S_1, first selfed generation; S_2, second, etc. (After Rogers & Ulmer, 1962.)

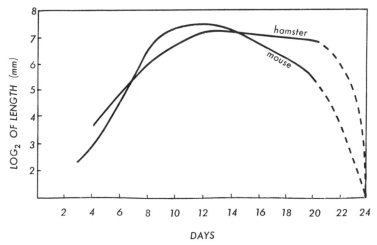

Fig. 59. Differential growth rates of *Hymenolepis nana* in the hamster and the mouse. (Modified from Schiller, 1959b.)

Growth Rate

Most investigations of growth have been concerned with length/weight/time or area/time studies and, with a few exceptions (Figs. 61, 66), little information is available on the change in chemical composition during development.

Before considering the growth rate, it is well to clarify what is implied by *growth* as distinct from *development* and *maturation*; for a more detailed discussion see Roberts,[329] and Clegg and Smyth.[72] A simplified definition of *growth*, which avoids the special problems of animals with few cell divisions (such as nematodes) is ' an increase in the total mass of protoplasm '. A generalised, non-biological definition is ' a relatively irreversible time-change in magnitude, of the measured dimension or function '.[329] *Development* is a combination of growth and differentiation, and is characterised by the production of progressively different groups of cells or tissues, which begin to synthesise different structural proteins and enzymes. It is widely recognised that cell and tissue differentiation are central problems in biology. Cestodes provide unusually interesting material for this field; for an adult cestode is essentially made up of a string of embryos, in organic continuity with one another, yet with increasing degrees of maturity; all developmental stages can, therefore, be studied in one organism. Again, several species of cestodes, e.g. *E. granulosus*, are capable of differentiation into either a cystic or strobilate phase, depending on the physico-chemical and nutritive conditions of their environment (Fig. 72). Since all these stages can now be developed *in vitro* (pp. 177–187) the value of a cestode as a biological model in the field of cell differentiation becomes apparent.

There are essentially two fundamentally different methods of expressing growth rate: (*a*) by measuring the ' absolute ' gain in a given dimension per unit time, or (*b*) by measuring the ' relative ' gain per unit time. Recent workers have used the term ' specific ' rather than ' relative ' (or ' percentage ') rate of growth, as it is usually thought to yield its information more easily. According to Medawar, ' it provides a record of the *multiplication* of living substance, for the integral quantity that is plotted against time is not size itself ($\int dW$) but the logarithm of the size, that is to say $\int dW/W$ '.[329]

Information on growth rates is available for *D. latum*;[419] *D. mansoni*;[445] *D. dendriticum*;[12] *H. diminuta*;[128, 329] *H. nana*;[367] *R. kashiwarensis*;[358] *H. taeniaeformis*;[178] *T. saginata*;[419] *E. granulosus*.[423]

An initial lag period in the growth rate has been reported in some species. Factors which appear to operate to produce this lag are, (*a*) the initial establishment in an unfavourable posterior region of the intestine, followed by a later migration forwards to a more favourable duodenal site, (e.g. *D. dendriticum*[12]) (*b*) an initial period, during which close contact with the mucosa (which is necessary in some species, e.g. *E. granulosus*[423]) is being established. Many other factors may also operate. A well known laboratory cestode which has an initial lag

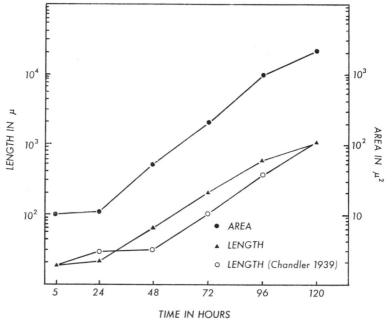

Fig. 60. Growth of *Hymenolepis diminuta* during the first five days in the final rat host; semi-log scale. (After Goodchild & Harrison, 1961.)

phase is *H. diminuta*, in which the lag period is about twenty-four hours, after which the growth rate rises sharply (Fig. 60). In this species there appears to be very little difference in growth rates measured using weight or area as parameters.

In *E. granulosus* growth as measured by increase in total nitrogen, lags for the first five days—a lag which is paralleled by the glycogen level (Fig. 61). A lag phase of about three days has also been reported in *D. mansoni*.[445] In contrast, the growth of *H. taeniaeformis* commences immediately on entering the small intestine[178]. The absence of a lag period in this species is attributed to the fact that initial establishment occurs in the small intestine, a nutritionally favourable site. In this species there appear to be two exponential phases of adult growth.

The first phase terminates on the eighteenth day after infection, with a doubling time of eight days.   Then follows a period of deceleration, and the growth patterns enter a second exponential phase with a doubling time of sixteen days;   the transition point between the two phases

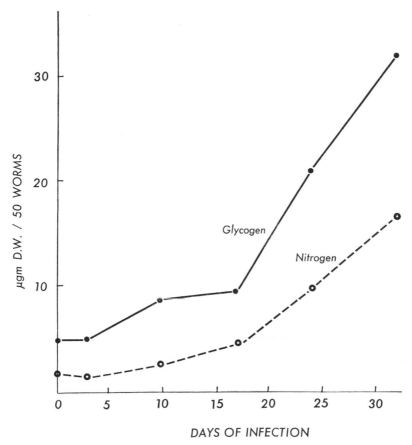

FIG. 61. Glycogen and nitrogen levels in *Echinococcus granulosus*.   (After Smyth & Miller, 1968.)

coincides approximately with the commencement of egg production, between the sixteenth and eighteenth day (Fig. 62).

A general slowing down in the growth rate after the onset of egg production is common in other species also, and may be attributed to the cessation of somatic growth in mature proglottids.

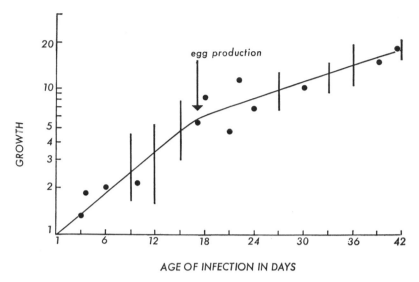

FIG. 62. Growth curve for adult phase of *Hydatigera* (*Taenia*) *taeniae-formis* in the cat measured on a logarithmic scale. Growth is calculated by expressing fresh weight of worm as multiple of fresh weight of larva strobila. (Modified from Hutchison, 1959.)

Strobilisation, Organogeny and Maturation

Induction of Strobilisation

With the exception of a few forms with progenetic plerocercoids (e.g. *Schistocephalus*), it is only within the definitive host intestine that cestode tissue develops in a strobilar direction. It can thus be concluded that this differentiation is induced by factors present in the intestinal environment. Any number of the known parameters of the intestine (Fig. 8) could act in this capacity. It is well recognised that in nematodes the high intestinal pCO_2 serves as a 'trigger' which switches the organism from the larval to the adult metabolism;[334] a similar mechanism may operate with some cestode species, possibly via CO_2 fixation. In general, however, the nature of the factors inducing strobilisation in cestodes is unknown. An exception is *Echinococcus*, in which it has been shown by *in vitro* experiments[423, 428, 430] that the contact of the rostellum with a suitable protein substrate induces strobilar growth (p. 182).

Presumably, such stimuli operate through sensory receptors (with which the scolex abounds), and in this respect it is interesting to note that neurosecretory material has been detected in the scolex of *H.*

diminuta (p. 20) during the stage of early differentiation but neither in the cysticercoid nor in the adult worm.[91a] This result would support the speculation (p. 184) that in *Echinococcus* the 'contact' stimulus mentioned above may operate via a neurosecretion which in turn induces the release of a 'strobilisation organiser' (Fig. 76).[430] Analysis of the factors inducing strobilar growth would appear to be a particularly fruitful field for future work.

Stages in Maturation

Organogeny and maturation involve the production of a large number of cells, the differentiation of these into organs, and the maturation of the gonads and associated structures. It is convenient to divide the process of maturation into a series of stages which can serve as recognisable criteria for assessing development. Identification of these stages has been of particular value in *in vitro* studies. Different workers have used slightly different criteria in cyclophyllidean and pseudophyllidean cestodes.[24-26, 430] The stages in cyclophyllid development as exemplified by *Echinococcus*, are shown in Fig. 63; pseudophyllid development is shown in Fig. 67.

Briefly, the stages in *Echinococcus* may be summarised as follows (Fig. 63):

Stage 0—Undeveloped Metacestode. This stage is represented by the evaginated, but undeveloped, metacestode.

Stage 1—Segmentation. The appearance of the first proglottid of the developing strobila represents a clearly recognisable stage of development. This stage is foreshadowed by the appearance of a clear protoplasmic area in the region where the partition separating the first segment from the scolex will later appear. The excretory canals also become markedly prominent about this time.

Stage 2—Appearance of Second Proglottid. This stage too, is clearly defined by the appearance of a second interproglottid partition.

Stage 3—Early Gametogeny. This stage is characterised by the appearance of testes in the most posterior proglottid.

Stage 4—Genital Pore Formation. This stage is characterised by the appearance of the lateral genital pore. Although in whole mount preparations the genital pore appears small and contracted, in the living worm it appears larger and is in a constant state of activity, opening and closing at intervals—an activity probably related to copulatory behaviour.

Stage 5—Late Gametogeny. This stage is characterised by maturation of the male and female genitalia. The presence of mature spermatozoa, as observed by microscopic examination, is required to confirm that development has reached this stage. Spermatogenesis may be examined by preparing routine aceto-orcein squashes, a technique particularly good for detecting cytological abnormalities.[24] The presence of spermatozoa

in cultured worms, however, is not sufficient to indicate that ' normal '
development has occurred.   To satisfy this criterion, spermatozoa must
be morphologically normal, show activity, and be present in quantities
comparable with those in worms matured *in vivo*.

Stage 6—Uterus Dilation.   This stage is characterised by the appearance of the uterus, which appears initially as a hollow thin-walled sac,
in the centre of the maturing proglottid.

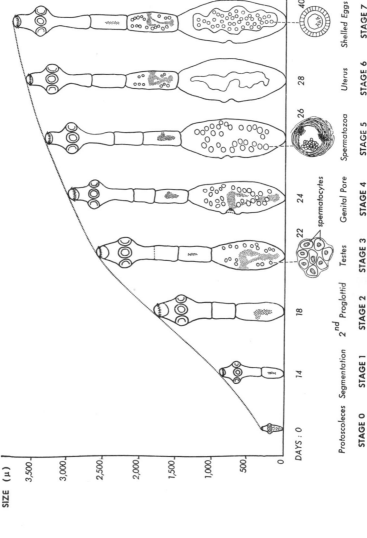

FIG. 63. Criteria for the development and maturation of *Echinococcus granulosus*. (After Smyth, Miller &
Howkins, 1967.)

Stage 7—*Oncosphere Formation*. This stage is characterised by the appearance in the uterus of embryonated eggs containing fully formed 6-hooked oncospheres. Microscopical examination is necessary to confirm that a hooked embryo is present and that such embryos are active.

Factors Affecting Maturation

The growth rate, the form of organogeny associated with it, and the onset of maturation are likely to be influenced by a number of factors related to the physiology of the host intestine; of these the following are probably the most important:

physico-chemical:	temperature, pH, pCO_2, pO_2, E_h.
biochemical:	composition of bile, concentration and ratio of amino acids.
morphological:	micromorphology of mucosa.
nutritional:	diet of host, especially regarding carbohydrate level.
immunological:	host species or strain.
hormonal:	sex of host.
behavioural:	whether host is stressed or normal.

The importance of the micromorphology of the gut has been considered earlier (p. 26). Of the remaining factors, only a few have been investigated, some of which are discussed below:

Influence of host species. It is difficult to separate the influence of host species *per se* (i.e. immunological influences) from influences due to physiological differences between host species. It has already been stressed (Fig. 59) that growth rates of a cestode species may vary in different hosts. It has also been shown, in *H. nana*, that the frequency of abnormal characteristics (such as two testes instead of three) varied markedly with host species (Table 37).

Influence of temperature. The influence of temperature has been shown to be of especial importance in the maturation of the pseudophyllidean genera *Schistocephalus*, *Ligula* and *Digramma*, which have cold-blooded intermediate hosts and warm-blooded definitive hosts. Thus, the plerocercoids of *Schistocephalus*, when cultured *in vitro* under suitable physiological conditions, reach maturity and produce fertile eggs[410] (p. 169). The threshold temperature, beneath which maturation will not occur, is in the region of 34°C.[409] From a detailed study of the effect of temperature on the growth rate and maturation of this species it has been speculated that the plerocercoid contains two enzyme systems, one controlling somatic growth with a peak efficiency near

TABLE 37

Frequency of occurrence of variant characteristics in Hymenolepis nana *according to host-species in which cestodes developed following direct and indirect experimental infections*
(Data from Schiller[369])

	Variant characteristic											
	Reduction in testes numbers						Sterility					
	Number of proglottids examined		Number with two testes		Percent with two testes		Number of proglottids examined		Number of sterile proglottids		Percent of proglottids sterile	
Host-species	Direct	Indirect	Direct	Indirect	Direct	Indirect	Direct	Indirect	Direct	Indirect	Direct	Indirect
Albino mouse	4,363	5,126	121	113	2·8	2·2	8,347	8,129	21	25	0·25	0·31
Albino hamster	6,972	7,640	216	221	3·1	2·9	5,947	5,773	30	32	0·50	0·55
Marmota monax	4,152	6,512	112	182	2·7	2·8	6,203	4,223	26	22	0·58	0·52
Sciurus carolinensis	6,112	6,302	305	334	5·0	5·3	6,682	6,282	88	95	1·40	1·50
Tamiasciurus hudsonicus	—	4,018	—	185	—	4·6	—	7,264	—	60	—	0·83
Glaucomys volans	2,123	2,094	104	98	4·9	4·7	3,417	3,537	36	35	1·10	1·00
Dipodomys merriami	991	1,756	24	40	2·4	2·3	2,050	2,068	15	16	0·75	0·77
Oryzomys palustris	4,297	3,912	120	109	2·8	2·8	4,496	3,610	12	10	0·27	0·28

23 °C, and another controlling genitalia maturation with a peak efficiency near 40°C.[394]   In the plerocercoid, synthesis of both somatic and genital tissue occur.   In the case of worms over 10 mg, a temperature over 34°C stimulates oogenesis, spermatogenesis and vitellogenesis to take place and presumably inhibits somatic growth (Fig. 64).[170]

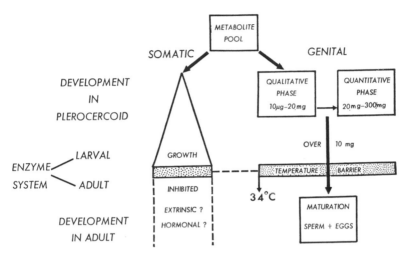

FIG. 64. Pattern of development in *Schistocephalus solidus* during the plerocercoid and adult phases. (Modified from Hopkins & McCaig, 1963.)

Influence of diet on growth.   Since cestodes are intestinal parasites, it is only to be expected that the nature of host diet will affect growth of the contained parasites.   The effect on the growth rate of cestodes, (especially *H. diminuta*)[240, 310–312, 315] of altering the carbohydrate or protein levels in the diet of the host has been examined earlier (Chapters 5, 6).   It was shown that the growth rate was markedly dependent on the carbohydrate level of the host diet, but virtually independent of the quantity or quality of protein.   Proglottid release is also influenced to some extent by the feeding habits of the host.[419]

Influence of worm load—the ' crowding effect '.   It has long been recognised that, in cestode infections the size of individual worms appeared to be inversely related to the number of worms present in the gut, a phenomenon known as the ' crowding effect '.   A number of attempts have been made to quantify this effect, and data are available for *H. nana*,[316] *H. diminuta*,[298, 304, 316, 329] *R. cesticillus*,[324] and *D. latum*.[281-2]

Competition for available carbohydrate appears to be the major factor concerned in the 'crowding effect'. Thus, when *single* strobila of *H. citelli* and *H. diminuta* were grown in the same host fed on an unlimited starch diet, both species were affected. *H. citelli* was affected

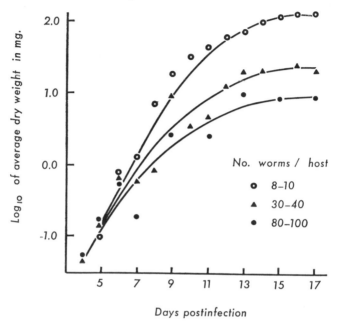

FIG. 65. The 'crowding' effect in *Hymenolepis diminuta*; growth measured in dry weight at different population densities. (After Roberts, 1961.)

proportionately more than *H. diminuta*, being reduced to 36% of its size when present alone (Table 38). Under carbohydrate deprivation (0·5 g starch/day) the size of *H. citelli* was not affected by the presence of *H. diminuta*, whereas *H. diminuta* was further reduced in size under these conditions. When 5–30 worms were grown in rats fed on a 'standard' starch diet, 'limited' starch or sucrose, a similar crowding effect was observed.

In *H. diminuta*, the relationship between weight and number of worms in an infection has been expressed by the general equation:

$$y = kx^n,$$

when $n = -1$, $xy = k$.

Except for the brief initial lag phase, growth in *H. diminuta* (Fig. 60) is most rapid during the first seven days; thereafter a phase of retardation sets in until patency at 16–17 days.[329]   The effects of population density become particularly apparent during this latter phase (Fig. 65). Although size and weight are affected by crowding, the onset time of maturation is not apparently affected by population size.   A study of the chemical embryology of the maturing *H. diminuta* showed that

TABLE 38

The interaction of Hymenolepis citelli *and* Hymenolepis diminuta *in hamsters given unlimited or restricted quantities of carbohydrate for eight days.   Data are expressed as mean ± standard error*

(Data from Read and Phifer[309])

Parasites in the individual host. (Single cysticercoids fed.)	Diet	Wet weight worm (mg.)		No. of Animals
		H. citelli	*H. diminuta*	
H. citelli	starch *ad lib.*	365·9±38·3	—	5
H. diminuta	starch *ad lib.*	—	734·5±58·0	4
H. citelli plus *H. diminuta*	starch *ad lib.*	134·5± 5·0	639·8±29·9	5
H. citelli	0·5g. starch/day	100·8±10·2	—	5
H. diminuta	0·5g. starch/day	—	363·6±14·7	4
H. citelli plus *H. diminuta*	0·5g. starch/day	107·4±15·1	269·9±21·8	4

crowding markedly affected the carbohydrate and lipid content of worms during development.[329]   In worms from small populations (fewer than 30 worms per host) the carbohydrate content rose from 20% to about 40%, but in higher populations only a marginal increase occurred.   In all populations (3–100 worms per host), a marked decrease in the total protein content occurred (from 60–70% to 30%), and similarly the phospholipid content fell from 10% to 3% (Fig. 66). The lipid content remained relatively constant.   Calculation of the heterauxetic rate constants relative to increase in dry weight showed that protein and phospholipid were bradyauxetic, carbohydrate was tachyauxetic with a tendency towards isoauxesis with increasing population size and lipids were bradyauxetic or isoauxetic with a tendency towards tachyauxesis with increased population.   These results with *H. diminuta* are in contrast with those found in another cyclophyllidean, *Hydatigera taeniaeformis*, in which the protein synthesis was shown to be isoauxetic and not bradyauxetic as in *H. diminuta*.[168]   This result was attributed to a fall in glycogen rather than to a faster rate of protein synthesis.

Since the ' crowding effect ' appears to have mainly a nutritional basis, it is not unexpected to find that cestode growth can be influenced by the presence of parasites other than cestodes.   Thus, the acanthocephalan *Moniliformis dubius* depresses the growth rate of *H. diminuta* in Holtzman rats[159, 160] but not in hamsters.[161]   Further evidence that the crowding effect in rats was related to competition for carbohydrate has been provided by the fact that this effect did not occur in rats injected with phlorizin, a drug which simulates diabetes and increases the availability of utilisable carbohydrate in the gut.

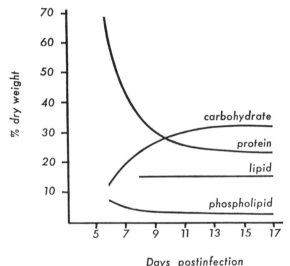

Days postinfection

FIG. 66. Relative changes in chemical composition of *Hymenolepis diminuta* at a population level of 3-5 worms per host. (After Roberts, 1961.)

Influence of hormones on growth.   Since the cestode metabolism is dependent on the host metabolism, and since the latter is influenced by the endocrine system, it is not unexpected that the hormonal activity of the host appears to have some influence on cestode growth and development.   Much of the evidence for this, however, is indirect and equivocal.   For example, it is known that several species of cestodes of fish, in the temperate zone, show correlation of season and maturation, the latter process taking place only in summer.

Examples of these are: *Proteocephalus filicollis* in *Gasterosteus aculeatus*; *Corallobothrium giganteum* and *C. fimbriatum* in *Ictalurus punctatus*; *Triaenophorus crassus*, *T. nodulosus* in *Esox lucius* and *Proteocephalus stizostethi* in *Stizostedion vitreum vitreum*[164].

Although these effects are generally attributed to rise in temperature, changes in the hormonal pattern, or other seasonal factors, such as changes in the food of the host, may be involved.   In *H. diminuta*, neither testosterone nor progesterone appears to be necessary for normal growth *in vivo* and the hormonal requirements may be related to the host diet, since growth is normal in male rats maintained on a vitamin-deficient diet, but stunted in female rats on the same diet.[22] Since *in vitro* experiments with *H. diminuta* have shown that maturation can be achieved in the absence of sex hormones,[370] it is clear that the hormone effect is due to an indirect effect on the metabolism of the host rather than to a direct effect on the worm.

Bile. There is no evidence that cestodes require bile in order to grow normally. Lack of bile (as in surgically altered rats) has been shown to markedly inhibit growth and egg-production in *H. diminuta*.[123, 124] That this is due to an effect on the host rather than on the parasite is shown by the fact that this species may be grown to maturity *in vitro* in the absence of bile (p. 173).

Influence of radiation. X-radiation at reasonable dose levels is well known to produce morphological abnormalities in living organisms, and cestodes are no exception. The effects of doses of X-rays or cobalt 60 in the region of 5 – 40,000 roentgens on the development of *H. nana* and *H. diminuta*, have been examined,[368, 459] and in *H. nana* no adult cestodes were obtained from eggs exposed to more than 30 000 R.[368] In *H. nana*, below the lethal level of radiation no abnormalities occurred which could not be found in normal (non-irradiated) worms. The X-irradiation merely made a given mutation more frequent, and, following the normal genetic pattern, the frequency of radiation tended to be proportional to the dose received. In *Hymenolepis microstoma*, it was found that worms damaged by radiation could recover, the damaged strobila being replaced by a normal one.[447] This recovery appeared to be related to the fact that, although the proglottid-forming region of the strobila was radiosensitive, the tissues of the neck region were radio-resistant.

10: *In Vitro* Cultivation of Cestodes

General Considerations

One of the most exciting developments in parasitology during the past decade has been the realisation that the nutritional and environmental requirements of cestodes can be sufficiently met by artificial systems, for development and maturation to take place outside the host. With metacestodes as initial culture material, a number of species have been cultured to maturity, or near maturity, *in vitro*.

In vitro techniques allow the nutrition, physiology and biochemistry of a parasite to be studied in isolation from the interacting physiology of the host; they are also of especial value in studying its immunological behaviour. Application of routine immunological techniques allow antibodies and antigens to be identified, but *in vitro* culture methods can often be used to demonstrate also which antigen-antibody reactions are *functional* (p. 216) in inhibiting development.

It is intended here to discuss only the general problems underlying *in vitro* culture and to deal with those organisms which have been cultured most successfully; early *in vitro* work has been reviewed elsewhere.[234, 316, 406, 417, 476] More recent work has been reviewed by Silverman,[389] Clegg and Smyth,[72] Hopkins,[166] Taylor and Baker.[450]

Terminology

A number of terms are in use to designate particular culture techniques. Thus, cultivation in the absence of any other organism (i.e. a 'pure' culture) is termed 'axenic' (Greek *a* = free from; *xenos* = stranger). A culture with another organism present is said to be 'monoxenic'; when more than one species are present, the term 'polyxenic' is used. The term '*in vitro*' (meaning literally 'in glass') has long been used to describe a culture involving a liquid or solid medium in a glass tube or similar container. An *in vitro* culture is not necessarily axenic, although it may be; the widespread use of antibiotics, for example, often permits the presence of micro-organisms in cultures at a level low enough not to interfere with the development of the parasite. For convenience, the more general term *in vitro* is used here.

Basic Problems of Cultivation

Cultivation of cestodes presents a number of problems, many of which are shared with other parasitic helminths such as nematodes and trematodes.[389, 422] Some problems, however, are unique to cestodes, particularly those related to the lack of an alimentary canal. Since adult cestodes normally inhabit intestinal sites, the chief stumbling-block to culture attempts in the past has been the initial establishment of sterility. Availability of antibiotics has eliminated this difficulty, and now there seems to be no reason why any species from any host site cannot be obtained in a sterile condition.

Once sterility is established, a number of other problems arise, the chief of which may be summarised as follows.

(*a*) The physico-chemical characteristics of the habitats of adult and larval cestodes are rather poorly known. Although the broad characteristics of the vertebrate alimentary canal are known (Chapter 3) little accurate information is available on the precise conditions in specific intestinal sites such as, for example, a crypt of Lieberkühn, in which the cestode scolex may be embedded. Data on tissue sites, such as the liver, muscle, body cavity, blood stream, brain, etc., are also limited. Information necessary to establish culture conditions would include data on the pH, pO_2, pCO_2, oxidation-reduction potential, amino-acid and sugar level, temperature, osmotic pressure and concentration levels of the common physiological ions (Fig. 8). Much of this kind of information is difficult to obtain, with accuracy, for any technique of measurement is itself likely to interfere with the very characteristics (e.g. pO_2), it is attempting to measure. Results from *in vitro* work, reviewed below, have shown that individual species may have very specific nutritional requirements, and what is satisfactory for one species may not be so for another, even though it utilises the same site in the same host. In this respect the pO_2, the oxidation-reduction potential (E_h) and the pH appear to be of particular importance.

(*b*) The nutritional materials available to cestodes in intestinal and tissue sites are complex and difficult to replace by defined media.

(*c*) The surface configuration of the intestine is usually elaborate and difficult to reproduce *in vitro*, and the reproduction of it is of especial importance with some species, e.g. *Echinococcus granulosus* (p. 180).

(d) In their natural habitat, the metabolic waste products of adult or larval cestodes are readily removed from the site of their production as a result of the natural circulation of body fluids. A successful *in vitro* method must similarly provide conditions which permit the rapid removal of toxic waste products.

(e) The complex nature of cestode life cycles, often involving three hosts, generally results in each stage having different nutritional requirements and requiring different physico-chemical conditions for development. Moreover, 'trigger stimuli' (p. 154) may be required at specific points in the life cycle before the organism can develop from one stage to another.

Criteria for Development

Before considering the so-called 'cultivation' methods, it is important to distinguish between conditions and media which permit mere *survival* and those which allow growth, development and maturation to occur. The term 'survival' is not easy to define with any precision, and even more difficult to measure *in vitro*. 'Survival' is here interpreted as implying merely the maintenance of an organism *in vitro* at a metabolic level sufficient to keep its cells and tissues alive, but not sufficient to allow growth and differentiation to occur in the case of metacestodes, or maturation of genitalia with the *continuous* production of normal sperm and eggs in the case of an adult worm.

In order to obtain an accurate assessment of these processes *in vitro*, it is essential to have a great deal of detailed information on the pattern of development and maturation in the natural host; this information should normally include morphological and cytological studies. Establishment of this pattern, related to a time scale, should therefore be the first step in an attempt at *in vitro* culture of any cestode species. Without such a pattern, it is impossible to assess accurately the degree of success of culture attempts. Unfortunately, the detailed developmental patterns *in vivo* are known for only a few cestodes, and are confined, for the most part, to commonly used experimental organisms such as *Hymenolepis*, *Schistocephalus*, *Ligula*, *Echinococcus*, and *Diphyllobothrium*.

The completion of normal embryonic development and maturation are clearly the only satisfactory criteria for development. Other criteria have been used, however, by some workers; these include[389] mobility and reaction to stimuli, size increase, physiological or biochemical criteria, such as utilisation of substrate and mitotic rate. Most of these are unsatisfactory for one reason or another. For example, a worm may show movement in culture long after its metabolic processes have ceased to function 'normally' (i.e. within the metabolic levels encountered *in vivo*). Again, even biochemical data have to be interpreted with caution. Thus, in a worm whose metabolism is inhibited by the conditions of cultivation, the carbohydrate reserves may remain at a relatively high level, on account of a depressed metabolism. However, these reserves may compare favourably with those of an organism which is metabolising normally but replenishing its reserves from the nutrients in the medium. The obvious means of distinguishing between these two diverse conditions is to relate biochemical data to morphogenesis, especially in relation to maturation and egg production.

Although there is some variation between different classes, the main criteria of development (p. 155) relate to segmentation, organogeny, gametogenesis and egg-shell formation (Figs. 63 and 67).

Species Used

Since adult cestodes are invariably coated with a mucus film containing microorganisms such as yeasts, bacteria and fungi, most workers have used metacestodes, which occur in sterile habitats, as initial culture material. Nevertheless, by use of antibiotics certain species of adult cestodes (e.g. *H. diminuta, E. granulosus*) may readily be cultured *in vitro* after removal from the definitive host, and maintained for long periods with egg production continuing at a level approaching the normal.[370, 427] Using metacestodes as initial material the following species have been cultured to maturity or near maturity, namely *H. nana, H. microstoma, H. diminuta*;[25, 26, 352a, 370, 393] *E. granulosus*;[423, 428, 430] *S. mansonoides*;[29] *S. solidus*;[405, 410, 415] *Ligula intestinalis*.[407, 412, 415]

Pseudophyllidea

General Comments

The Pseudophyllidea contain many well-known species which infect birds and mammals and whose plerocercoids occur in cold-blooded vertebrates, especially fish. Several genera are progenetic, e.g. *Schistocephalus, Ligula, Digramma*; and furthermore, the larvae contain sufficient carbohydrate and protein reserves to satisfy the energy and synthetic requirements of maturation. Such larvae provided useful experimental models for early work in this field, as maturation could be achieved *in vitro* once the appropriate environmental conditions were provided. Although experiments with such larvae did not initially provide much information on their nutritional requirements, they provided much basic data on the physico-chemical conditions under which maturation and fertilisation could take place. Once these were

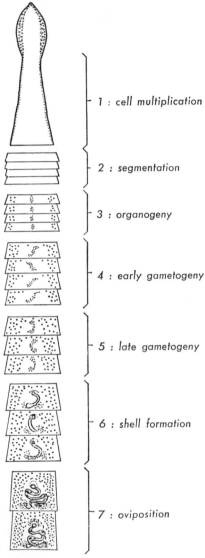

FIG. 67. Developmental stages of a cestode as exemplified by *Diphyllobothrium* sp. (After Smyth, 1959.)

determined, it was possible to carry out a range of cytological and biochemical investigations.

Culture of Progenetic Plerocercoids to Adults

Schistocephalus solidus. The progenetic plerocercoids of this species already contain the anlagen of the genitalia while still within the fish host. Maturation thus only involves differentiation from stage 4 to stage 7 (Fig. 67), a process which takes only thirty-six hours in the intestine of the bird host.[171] By painting the surface of the fish host with an antiseptic solution (such as iodine in 90% alcohol), it is a relatively simple matter to remove a plerocercoid in a sterile condition and transfer it to a receptacle containing culture media. Early experiments[405] established that worms became sexually mature adults, even in non-nutrient saline, when incubated at bird body temperature (40°C). Eggs produced in these preliminary experiments were infertile, and histological examination revealed that (a) spermatozoa had not reached the receptaculum seminis, (b) the testes showed some cytological abnormalities. Subsequent work showed that for normal maturation and fertilisation, resulting in fertile egg production, to occur *in vitro*, the following conditions were necessary:[410, 415]

(i) use of highly buffered media to counteract the toxic effect of acidic metabolic products;

(ii) cultivation under anaerobic conditions or at an O_2 tension sufficiently low to prevent premature oxidation of the egg-shell precursors (p. 113) in the vitellaria;

(iii) compression within cellulose (dialysis) tubing to assure that insemination and fertilisation take place.

(iv) gentle agitation of culture media to assist diffusion of waste metabolites.

To establish these conditions and to simplify culture procedures, a tube with a ground glass assembly was developed (Fig. 68). Plerocercoids, cultured in a medium of horse serum within the cellulose tube of this system, produced eggs with up to 88% fertility.[415] Surface apposition by compression within the cellulose tubing (= an artificial 'gut') is essential for insemination, and in worms so cultured the receptaculum seminis is filled with spermatozoa. In contrast, in worms cultured free in the media i.e. without compression, the receptacula are empty and the eggs infertile.

Ligula intestinalis. The progenetic plerocercoids of *Ligula intestinalis* also may be brought to maturity *in vitro* by a technique similar to that described above for *Schistocephalus*.[14, 407, 415]

Culture of Undifferentiated Plerocercoids

Unlike the above progenetic species, the majority of pseudophyllidean plerocercoids are undifferentiated morphologically, and must undergo considerable growth and differentiation before sexual maturity can be achieved. This represents a level of growth comparable to that required for a cyclophyllidean to develop from a cysticercoid to an adult worm.

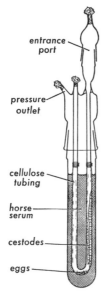

FIG. 68. Culture tube used for permitting *Schistocephalus solidus* to undergo impregnation during maturation. Note that fertile eggs are only produced by worms compressed within the cellulose tubing. (After Smyth, 1959.)

Diphyllobothrium spp. Plerocercoid larvae of *Diphyllobothrium* can survive in simple culture media, such as serum or broth, for periods of up to ten days.[415] Cultivation of such forms is difficult on account of the length of the strobila and the tendency of plerocercoids to tie themselves in knots. Attempts to overcome this difficulty by culturing plerocercoid fragments, instead of whole worms, using a duck embryo extract medium with a gas phase of air, led to partial success.[414-5] Fragments became segmented by the second day, developed genital anlagen by the third day and by the sixth day had become differentiated into miniature proglottids, some 1/5–1/10 the normal size, which contained a cirrus, uterus, ovary primordia and testes with spermatozoa.[415] Further cultivation (seven or eight days) resulted in autolysis—an effect probably due to the stage of intense protein synthesis related to egg formation. Addition of various supplements failed to improve development. Such early experiments left many factors—especially the gas phase—uncontrolled.

Spirometra mansonoides. More successful results were obtained with *S. mansonoides*[29] using a technique (described in further detail: p. 173) which had proved successful in the culture of cyclophyllidean cestodes. Starting with plerocercoids, which themselves had been cultured from procercoids *in vitro* (see below), and a complex culture medium (No. 115) a gas phase of 5% or 10% CO_2 in N_2, the plerocercoid of this species has been cultured through to early segmentation. The growth process involved scolex differentiation, shedding of the larval body, growth and early segmentation. Successful cultivation occurred only after plerocercoids had been evaginated (using bile solution), so that like *Echinococcus* (see p. 182) evagination may serve as a trigger stimulus, without which differentiation cannot occur. Oxygen appeared to be toxic to these worms in culture.

Culture of Coracidia to Procercoids

Some attempts to cultivate an oncosphere to a procercoid have been made with *Schistocephalus solidus*. It is relatively easy to obtain sterile eggs of this species, either by maturing the plerocercoid *in vitro* using the technique described earlier (p. 169), or by washing, in antibiotics, faecal eggs from a bird host. When eggs are allowed to embryonate and hatch in sterile oxygenated water, sterile coracidia are obtained.[412] Attempts to grow coracidia to procercoids, by using a variety of media, however, have proved unsuccessful, and this stage has so far defied cultivation for any pseudophyllidean species.

Culture of Procercoids to Plerocercoids

Spirometra mansonoides. Mueller[253-255, 262-3] in a series of detailed studies has developed a number of elegant techniques for obtaining procercoids of *S. mansonoides* in a sterile condition and subsequently cultivating them *in vitro* to infective plerocercoids.

For the detailed techniques, the original papers should be consulted. The method for embryonation and for hatching large quantities of eggs, basically consists of using 500 ml Erlenmeyer flasks containing concentrated suspensions of eggs obtained from cat faeces. The whole is shaken continuously, except for a short break of 1 min. every hour, and the water is changed frequently to avoid build-up of bacterial growth; if this does occur, it can be kept down by the addition of a few drops of iodine. Mass hatching of embryonated eggs occurs in strong sunlight, and the released coracidia readily infect the late nauplii and early copepod stages of *Cyclops vernalis*.[254] In 7–10 days the procercoids become infective to the cat host.

The basis of obtaining procercoids in sterile culture was the observation[254] that under the influence of heat, procercoids forced themselves out of infected copepods and may be harvested in a small modified Baermann apparatus (Fig. 69) adapted for obtaining sterile cultures.

Large numbers of procercoids were harvested by these methods and used as basic material for subsequent culture to the plerocercoid stage.

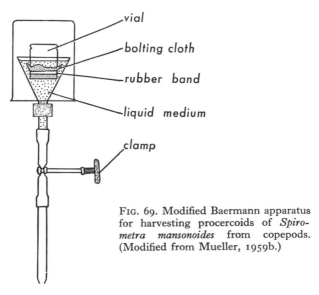

FIG. 69. Modified Baermann apparatus for harvesting procercoids of *Spirometra mansonoides* from copepods. (Modified from Mueller, 1959b.)

This was carried out in a liquid phase of Parker 199 + 10% calf serum + chick embryo extract (6 ml. 199 + CS to 1·5 ml. CEE) using a roller tube technique.[255, 262]

A remarkable degree of growth was obtained by this method, the worms almost doubling their size every twenty-four hours for the first week. Later, growth slowed down but a length of 20 mm was reached in thirty days—a rate of growth which compared favourably with that in the mouse host—and plerocercoids up to 30 mm were obtained in nine weeks. These plerocercoids were infective to cats and grew to mature *S. mansonoides*. A feature of plerocercoids cultured in mouse serum was the appearance of precipitates around the head and neck of the worm (Plate IV, A). This undoubtedly represents an immunological effect, and may be due to the use of non-inactivated serum; it closely resembles an effect noted in *Echinococcus in vitro* (p. 208; Plate IV, D.).

Schistocephalus solidus. The plerocercoids of *S. solidus*, which ranged from 2 to 200 mg in the body cavity of the stickleback *Gasterosteus aculeatus*, have been grown in a relatively simple medium.[233] In a liquid phase of 25% horse serum, 0·5% yeast extract, 0·65%

glucose and Hank's saline at $21°C$, and pH 7·1, and a gas phase of 5% CO_2 in air, dry weight-increases of up to 500% were recorded in eight days. Worms cultured for this period were able to mature when incubated at $40°C$ (p. 169). Growth during the next eight-day period was only 50–70% of the predicted rate and, by the end of the third period of eight days, had virtually stopped. A nutritional deficiency in the medium may have been responsible; but ultrastructure studies also revealed the presence of a thin layer of material of unknown origin, deposited over the microtriches of the tegument; this layer may have inhibited uptake of metabolites. This reaction may prove to be a common problem in cestode culture work and—as in *Echinococcus* (p. 210)—may represent a precipitate due to the presence of a non-specific antibody in the serum.

Cyclophyllidea

Many cyclophyllidean metacestodes—like pseudophyllidean plerocercoids—will ' survive ' in quite simple media, such as balanced saline plus glucose, for long periods without undergoing further development. Much of the early work, which was rather uncritical and empirical, has been reviewed elsewhere[406, 417] and will not be discussed further here. The major advances have been made by using *Hymenolepis*, *Echinococcus* and *Taenia* as models.

Hymenolepis *spp.*

Early experiments with this species[371] came very near to success. Adult worms were removed from the rat host, and the scolex and a small portion of the ' neck ' severed from the strobila. Best growth occurred in 50% horse serum plus a cestode tissue extract in roller tubes, and resulted in strobilisation; as many as 130 segments were formed, some having gonad differentiation. The gas phase was not stated.

Other early experiments with *H. diminuta* and *H. nana* met with little success.[448] Excysted larvae of these species from beetles were cultured in Parker 199 supplemented with serum and amino acids. Some growth occurred in *H. nana* in media to which mouse extract had been added.

Successful culture of both *H. diminuta* and *H. nana* was finally achieved by Berntzen,[25, 26] a result which represented a remarkable technical achievement. His method differed from those of earlier workers in that (*a*) it involved a continuous flow apparatus (Fig. 70) and (*b*) it utilised an extremely complex synthetic medium. The gas phase originally utilised was not stated, but presumably CO_2 was available. There is some doubt as to the exact composition of the complex liquid medium used, as unfortunately other workers have not succeeded in preparing it according to the instructions published. With this continuous flow method, cysticercoids were grown to sexually mature adults showing normal segmentation and well-developed gonads, and these eventually developed gravid proglottids with oncospheres.

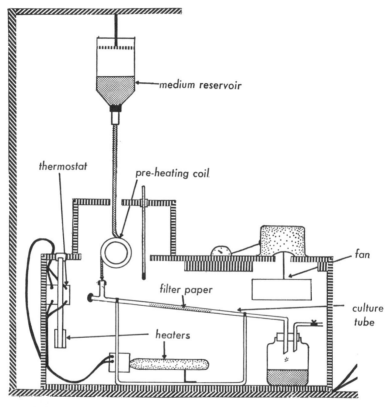

FIG. 70. Continuous flow apparatus, originally used for successful *in vitro* cultivation of *Hymenolepis diminuta*. (After Berntzen, 1961.)

Moreover, worms matured *in vitro* in a period of fifteen days—close to that required *in vivo* (thirteen days).

Subsequently, *H. nana* was grown to maturity *in vitro* by the same worker using a modified re-circulation technique—which utilised less medium (Fig. 71), a complex (largely synthetic) liquid phase (Medium 101 and 102), and a gas phase of 5% CO_2 in N_2.[26, 27] *H. microstoma* has also been grown to near maturity.[352a]

The success of this method appeared at first sight to be due to the facts that (*a*) the medium used contained a wide range of metabolites known to occur in cellular metabolism, (*b*) the medium was continually flowing so that the worms were being continually exposed to new supplies of metabolites and at the same time waste metabolic products were being continually swept away, (*c*) the gas phase was (apparently?)

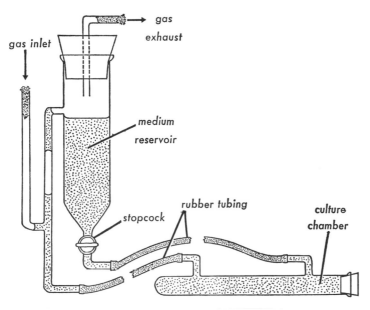

FIG. 71. A single recirculating unit used for the successful culti-vation of *Hymenolepis nana*. (Modified from Berntzen, 1962.)

controlled, and (*d*) the oxidation-reduction potential was also controlled, at least initially.

Although the initial cultivation of *H. diminuta* and *H. nana* repre-sented a major step forward in *in vitro* culture technique, some of the conclusions reached[25-27] as a result of these experiments are open to question on the grounds of being equivocal and sometimes based (apparently) on the results of a single experiment. Thus, although it was initially shown[26] that *H. nana* could reach maturity in an anaerobic gas phase of 5% CO_2 in N_2, it was later stated[27] that *no* growth occurred with this gas phase, and that an *aerobic* phase of 5% O_2 (+5% CO_2 in N_2) was essential. A critical analysis of Berntzen's results has been made by Hopkins[166] and, until more precise and less conflicting evidence is presented, it must be concluded that the precise growth requirements of *Hymenolepis* spp. have yet to be determined.

The requirements of both *H. diminuta* and *H. nana* may, however, prove to be simpler than the above results suggest, for cysticercoids of these species have since been cultured in much simpler systems without continuous flowing media.[370, 393] *H. diminuta* has been grown in a diphasic medium consisting of a blood-agar base (NNN) simply overlaid with Hank's balanced saline solution and a gas phase of 3% CO_2 in N_2.[370] Worms were initially cultured in flasks in a Dubnoff metabolic shaking incubator, and after six days were transferred to petri dishes with the same media; additional glucose was added from time to time and further transfers made. Gravid worms were produced by this method, and the oncospheres produced were infective to beetles and grew to normal worms in rats. Worms developed *in vitro* differed from *in vivo* worms in that: (a) the time required to reach maturity was twenty-four days compared with thirteen days required in the rat; (b) the worms were 'miniature' in size compared with those grown in a rat; (c) in gravid worms, many proglottids were sterile, although containing spermatozoa and oocytes—a result probably due to failure of insemination to take place. All these deviations from 'normal' development are reminiscent of those obtained with other species. Thus, fragments of *Diphyllobothrium* produced miniature proglottids *in vitro* (p. 170), and *Echinococcus* takes twice as long to mature *in vitro* and, moreover, fails to become inseminated (p. 184).

TABLE 39

Liver-extract medium which supports growth of Hymenolepis nana *cysticercoids to egg-producing adults in fourteen days* (*medium changed every three days*)
(Data from Sinha & Hopkins [393])

30% Horse serum
0·3% Glucose
0·5% Yeast extract
40% Hanks's saline
10% Rat liver extract$_{20}$

Antibiotics (100 i.u. Sodium Penicillin G+100 μg
Streptomycin sulphate (Crystamycin-Glaxo)/ml
of medium
$NaHCO_3$ (1·4%)+NaOH (0·2M)
pH 7·2 Gas 95% N_2+5% CO_2 Roller tubes at 37°

H. nana similarly has been grown to maturity in a simple medium containing horse serum, glucose, yeast extract, Hank's saline, rat liver extract and antibiotics (Table 39) in a gas phase of 5% CO_2 in N_2.[393] Using this medium in a roller tube technique, *H. nana* has been grown to maturity in twelve days—a time which closely approximates that *in vivo*. The difficulties of *in vitro* work are well illustrated by the fact that in one series of experiments with *H. nana*, out of six batches of yeast extract used (from different manufacturers) only three supported growth.[166] The factors in the yeast extract or liver extract which are essential for growth have not yet been identified.

Echinococcus *spp.*: *Cystic Differentiation*

General problems. The hydatid organism, *Echinococcus granulosus*, is a species which presents particularly interesting problems of morphogenesis; but, since its maturation period is 35–40 days *in vivo*, it is an exceptionally tedious experimental organism to work with. The closely related *E. multilocularis* (probably a ' strain ' of *E. granulosus*) develops more rapidly (30 days).

The larval stages (protoscoleces) in the hydatid cyst are remarkable for having the potential of differentiating in one of two directions, depending on their location within the host. Thus, when a hydatid cyst is eaten by a dog, the freed protoscoleces develop into adult strobilated tapeworms in the duodenum. On the other hand, if a hydatid cyst ruptures while still within the intermediate host (e.g. sheep, man), each of the released protoscoleces is capable of differentiating into a new hydatid cyst, which in turn develops protoscoleces, should it reach a suitable tissue site (i.e. secondary hydatidosis develops). This represents a degree of heterogeneous morphogenesis exceptional in a metazoan organism, and makes *Echinococcus* an unusual model for the study of cell differentiation.[423a] It is clear that factors present in the intestinal and tissue environments are responsible for initiating differentiation in these two directions. Elucidation of these factors— especially those inducing strobilisation—has been a major problem in *in vitro* work and the nature of some of the controlling factors involved have only recently become apparent.[423, 423a, 428, 430]

Growth pattern of the protoscolex. When cultured *in vitro*, a protoscolex can develop into a variety of different forms,[423] and it is important to appreciate the interrelationships between these before considering the more general problems of cystic or strobilar growth (Fig. 72).

The following forms have been identified :

Unevaginated protoscolex (Fig. 72A). The protoscolex remains undifferentiated as in a hydatid cyst.

Posterior bladder type (Fig. 72C). A small ' bladder '[418] or ' vesicle '[492] develops in the posterior region of an unevaginated protoscolex, apparently at the original site of attachment to the brood capsule wall ; this bladder eventually secretes a laminated envelope (see below) and becomes a miniature hydatid cyst.

Vesicular type (Fig. 72B). A protoscolex swells and becomes ' vesicular ' ; in the early stages the organism takes on a ' cottage-loaf '

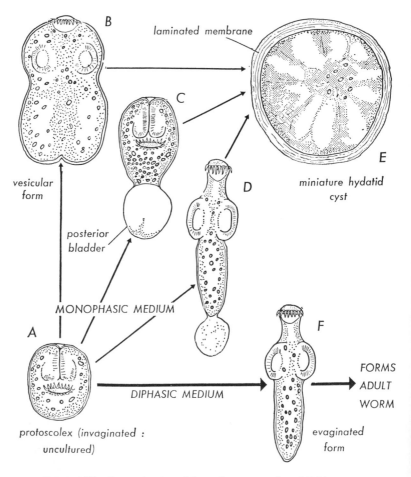

laminated membrane

B

C

E

vesicular form

miniature hydatid cyst

D

posterior bladder

MONOPHASIC MEDIUM

A

F

DIPHASIC MEDIUM

FORMS
ADULT
WORM

protoscolex (invaginated : uncultured)

evaginated form

FIG. 72. The forms developed from the protoscolex of *Echinococcus granulosus in vitro.* (After Smyth, 1967.)

shape. This type also secretes a laminated envelope and becomes a miniature cyst (*Fig.* 72E).

Evaginated protoscolex (Fig. 72F). When the scolex of a protoscolex evaginates, it results in an elongated organism which shows marked sucker and rostellum activity. This type normally develops into a strobilated adult worm.

Evaginated protoscolex with posterior bladder (*Fig.* 72D). This form appears to arise from a posterior bladder type, which becomes evaginated when the posterior bladder is in an early stage of development.

The relation of these culture types to cystic and strobilar development is discussed further below.

Cultivation of cystic stages. Under this heading are included attempts to cultivate the strobilate stage which were unsuccessful and which resulted in cystic development. Culture attempts to date have utilised hydatid cyst material—either pieces of germinal membrane or free protoscoleces.

Cystic E. multilocularis. The cystic stage of this species has proved more amenable to culture than *E. granulosus.* Fragments of germinal membrane have been grown in a basic medium of 40% ascitic fluid in Hank's saline plus HeLa cells and nutrients such as vole embryo extract; but unfortunately, full details of the technique have not been provided.[295] In these cultures, tissues proliferated and produced vesicles after 29 days culture; by 55 days some 20 protoscoleces were present in vesicles. Vesicles were shown to be infective to voles (the natural intermediate host) when injected into the body cavity. Other *in vitro* experiments utilising protoscoleces, separate vesicles, and minced tissues of the same species also resulted in protoscolex formation.[225] In a medium of Parker 199 supplemented with cotton rat (*Sigmodon hispidus*) embryo extract, bovine serum and lactalbumin hydrolysate, vesicles developed after 38 days, a laminated membrane in 54 days and protoscoleces after 99 days. The viability of these protoscoleces were proved by the development of cysts after intraperitoneal inoculation of cotton rats.

Less successful results were obtained with a basic medium of 0·5% lactalbumin hydrolysate in Hank's saline reinforced with various nutrients such as bovine serum, bile and liver extracts, in which only infertile cysts were formed.[492] These cysts were formed by two routes—as in *E. granulosus*—(a) by the protoscoleces becoming vesicular (Fig. 72B) and eventually secreting a *laminated membrane*—an envelope characteristic of a hydatid cyst, and (b) by protoscoleces which formed posterior bladders (Fig. 72C). In some cases, germinal cells, similar to those found in the early formation of a brood capsule, were formed; fully formed protoscoleces, however, were not produced.

Cystic E. granulosus. Early workers attempted the cultivation of protoscoleces of *E. granulosus* using a variety of media such as Parker 199 plus hydatid fluid, various sera and embryo extracts, after treatment with pepsin and a trypsin-pancreatin-bile mixture (to eliminate dead material).[418] Results were almost identical to those described above for *E. multilocularis*, i.e. protoscoleces formed small hydatid vesicles either by becoming vesicular or by forming posterior bladders (Figs. 72B; 72C). In both cases a laminated envelope was secreted; this was found to be strongly PAS-positive and appeared to be histologically identical with the mucopolysaccharide laminated layer of a hydatid cyst. It is interesting to note that this material has been found to be immunologically identical with the human blood group substance P, since (*a*) the medium in which protoscoleces were cultured became strongly positive for anti-P-inhibiting substance and (*b*) a protoscolex secreting a laminated membrane *in vitro* fluoresces when treated with fluorescent anti-P-serum.[431]

Other workers attempting *in vitro* culture using similar types of media obtained almost identical results[280] although in one case[135a] no laminated membrane appeared to be formed *in vitro*. This latter anomalous result may be due to the absence of some factor from the culture medium used, and it may indeed provide some clue as to the mechanism of laminated membrane formation.

Factors controlling vesicular (cystic) differentiation. A feature of the experiments described above is the fact that *in vitro* cultured worms sometimes become swollen or vesicular and eventually formed miniature hydatid cysts (Fig. 72E). The question naturally arises: What factors control differentiation in a vesicular direction? The effect of some physical factors on vesicularisation *in vitro* has been examined.[423,429, 473] These results at first appeared somewhat equivocal in that such varying factors as a high or low oxygen tension or a high pH ($>8\cdot0$) or low pH ($<5\cdot0$) induced vesicularisation. It was then realised that all these characteristics had one point in common—they were all ' abnormal ' relative to the conditions in the gut.[423] It was thus concluded that probably many, or perhaps any, *abnormal* condition induced a protoscolex to differentiate in a vesicular direction. Since a vesicular protoscolex secretes a laminated envelope, and, in fact, develops into a miniature hydatid cyst, the process of vesicularisation can be considered to represent a protective mechanism when viewed against the life cycle of the worm.

Echinococcus *spp.*: in vitro *differentiation of the strobilar stages*

Preliminary experiments. Determination of the factors which control the development of a protoscolex in a strobilar direction has been one of the most fascinating problems in *in vitro* studies. All early culture attempts resulted in cystic development. However, two groups of workers,[225, 473] utilising mainly *E. multilocularis*, obtained some degree of strobilisation. One series of experiments[473] utilised some forty-six, mainly complex, media (based on Morgan's M 150 medium and Parker's CMRL–1066) and obtained a few strobilated worms, but no genitalia development. One segmented worm was collected from a culture tube that had been lined with filter paper— a significant point, in view of the importance of the presence of a supporting surface, demonstrated later and discussed below. The precise conditions under which this result was obtained were not,

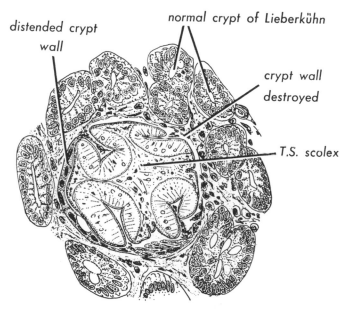

distended crypt wall

normal crypt of Lieberkühn

crypt wall destroyed

T.S. scolex

FIG. 73. T.S. crypt of Lieberkühn in the duodenum of a dog infected with *Echinococcus granulosus*. Note the extreme stretching and flattening of the crypt wall. (Original.)

however, clarified by these workers or confirmed by further work. A similar result was obtained by Lukashenko,[225] who reported development in some media of strobila with two or three segments, but no *genitalia development* took place.

Development to sexual maturity. The general failure of the more usual culture procedures to induce growth in a strobilar direction led to the conclusion that some unsuspected and unusual requirement was missing from the culture conditions provided. This led to the re-examination of the conditions under which an adult, strobilated worm lives and grows *in vivo* while attached to the intestinal mucosa—

an examination which ultimately provided the clue to the determination of the factors controlling strobilate development and led to the development of a technique which made this possible *in vitro*.[423, 428, 430]

Briefly, it was found that within the small intestine of a dog, *E. granulosus* penetrates to the base of the villi and lies with each sucker drawing a plug of epithelium into its cavity; the everted and extended rostellum of a worm normally penetrates a crypt of Lieberkühn (Fig. 12), stretching the epithelium of the crypt so that it becomes a thin layer of flattened cells (Fig. 73); occasionally, this layer is found

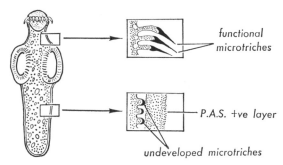

FIG. 74. *Echinococcus granulosus*—evaginated protoscolex showing presence of fully formed microtriches in the rostellar region only. (After Smyth, 1967.)

ruptured. Furthermore, the rostellar tip contains gland cells which secrete externally after about 20 days growth (Fig. 12). Consideration of these led to the conclusion that contact of the scolex with the cells of the mucosa was so close that perhaps it could be regarded as more of a tissue parasite than an intestinal one, at least during the early stages of establishment. If this hypothesis was sound, the organism could be expected to absorb directly through its contact with the mucosa. In other words, the scolex of *Echinococcus* could be regarded as being essentially *placental* in nature. These speculations were reinforced by investigations on the ultrastructure of the tegument (Fig. 74) which showed that, although the evaginated region of the protoscolex possessed microtriches (p. 9) these were missing from the region posterior to the suckers. This latter region was covered in a dense layer of mucopolysaccharide (PAS-positive), beneath which occurred what appeared to be undeveloped microtriches (Fig. 74). This led to the speculation that the requirement missing from the *in vitro* system was a solid substrate which could act both as a supporting surface and as one from which nutrient could be obtained.

Experiments have shown that this general hypothesis appears to hold. When protoscoleces were evaginated by treating with pepsin followed by a trypsin-pancreatin bile mixture (see p. 145) and cultured in a diphasic medium, the general pattern of growth *in vitro* proceeded in a strobilar direction.[423, 428]

The first culture system that was successful (Fig. 75D) consisted of a culture bottle containing a solid base of coagulated bovine or

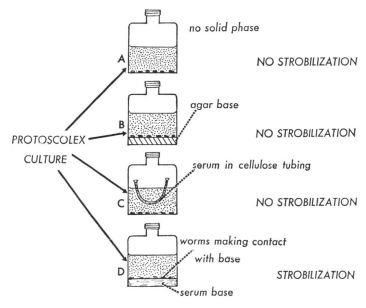

FIG. 75. Demonstration of the importance of contact with a protein substrate in the strobilar development of *Echinococcus granulosus in vitro*. Strobilisation only occurs in culture D. (After Smyth, Howkins & Barton, 1966.)

canine serum, into which a series of small holes or grooves were made with a fine pipette. The whole was covered with a liquid phase of Parker 199+20% hydatid fluid; a gas phase of 8·8% O_2+5% CO_2 in N_2 was initially used.[428] In this diphasic system, protoscoleces which were evaginated remained so, became visibly elongated, and eventually segmented. When the liquid phase was replaced by Parker 858+20% hydatid fluid and the gas phase changed to 10% O_2+5% CO_2 in N_2, worms grew to the three-segmented stage, in which both male and female genitalia developed to maturity; oogenesis occurred and large numbers of spermatozoa were obtained.[423, 430]

However, embryonated eggs did not form in cultured worms.

Histological examination revealed that the receptaculum seminis was empty—indicating that insemination (and consequently, fertilisation) had not taken place. This result is reminiscent of early experiments with the maturation of *Schistocephalus* (p. 169), in which failure to become inseminated *in vitro* was overcome by compressing during culture with semi-permeable cellulose tubing (Fig. 68). This result suggests that some physical requirement (such as compression) for insemination was lacking in the culture system used for *Echinococcus*. Nevertheless, since the eggs of this particular species are highly infective to man, the fact that an egg-less mature worm is produced is somewhat of an advantage—it means that the physiology of the mature stages can be examined without danger of infection.

These results clearly indicate that the presence of a solid base in some way stimulates growth in a strobilar direction. This naturally raises the fundamental question: What is the nature of this stimulus? Is the solid serum base successful in inducing strobilisation because it merely provides a ' surface ', which in turn induces a nervous stimulus by contact? If this hypothesis were true, any surface of similar consistency (e.g. agar) should induce the ' strobilisation stimulus '. Again, it could be asked: Are essential growth factors merely released into the medium by digestion of the surface of the host tissue—perhaps by ' membrane digestion ' (p. 90), and subsequently absorbed by the parasite?

If such a digestion process occurs, in or at the interface, are these released materials themselves essential for strobilisation, or do they produce a stimulus, perhaps via neurosecretion (p. 20) which releases an ' organiser ', which in turn initiates strobilisation (Fig. 76)?

It has been shown that in *Echinococcus* the microtriches are covered in what appear to be ' secretory ' membranes (Fig. 4), and it may be that in this species these are able to function properly only when in close contact with a suitable substrate.

The experiment illustrated in Fig. 75 tested some of these hypotheses; in summary, it consisted of the following cultures:

Culture Series A.   Liquid phase only—no solid base.
Culture Series B.   Agar base+liquid phase.
Culture Series C.   Solid serum base confined within cellulose tubing+liquid phase.
Culture Series D.   Solid serum base+liquid phase.

Strobilisation occurred only in cultures of Series D, i.e. those with a solid serum base (Fig. 75D). In all the other cultures (Series A, B, C), organisms became vesicular or formed posterior bladders and either eventually gave rise to miniature cysts (as in Fig. 72E) or died.

FIG. 76. Comparison of the protoscolex of *Echinococcus granulosus* in a hydatid cyst and, after evagination, in the dog gut. In the latter position, the exposed microtriches make contact with the protein surface and the cestode cells are stimulated to differentiate in a strobilar direction. It is speculated that an 'organiser' is involved, the release of which may be initiated via a neurosecretion. (After Smyth, Miller & Howkins, 1967.)

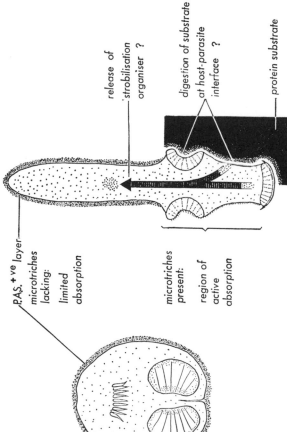

release of
'strobilisation
organiser ?

digestion of substrate
at host-parasite
interface ?

protein substrate

IN DOG GUT

P.A.S. +ve layer
microtriches
lacking:
limited
absorption

microtriches
present:
region of
active
absorption

IN HYDATID CYST

Moreover, only in Series D did the worms retain their ' activity '—
a vigorous muscular movement of suckers, rostellum and strobila.
In the absence of an ' exposed ' solid serum base (e.g. even with the
serum confined with cellulose tubing) this activity gradually fell off
until it ceased altogether, after which the cystic stage of development
ensued (Fig. 77).   This appeared to prove unequivocally that actual

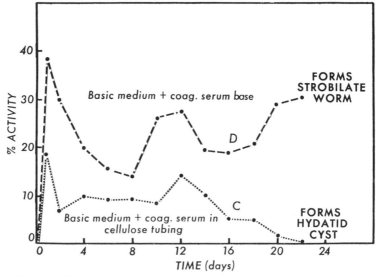

FIG. 77. Activity of *Echinococcus granulosus* protoscoleces *in vitro* in
culture vessels containing D, a diphasic medium with an exposed coagulated serum base, and C, a similar medium in which the serum base is
confined within a cellulose tubing so that worm/substrate contact is
prevented.   Strobilate worms only form in culture D (see Fig. 75).   (After
Smyth, 1967.)

contact of an evaginated worm with a nutritive base was necessary.
Whether the initial strobilisation stimulus is nutritive or nervous or
both, has yet to be determined.   The view that digestive enzymes are
released at the interface is further demonstrated by the fact that when
Echinococcus is cultured in a continuous flow system similar to that
utilised for *H. nana*—*even on a solid substrate*—*no* strobilar growth
occurs.[429]   This suggests that the enzyme(?) secreted is being swept
away from the microthrix surface.   If, however, the medium in contact
with the solid substrate and worm is allowed to remain undisturbed,
as in the ' stationary ' lift (Fig. 78), and further medium circulated
inside a semi-permeable cellulose tubing (through which nutrient,
gaseous and waste material exchange could take place), excellent growth

to the 3-strobilar stage takes place.[429] This has proved to be the most satisfactory culture technique to date.

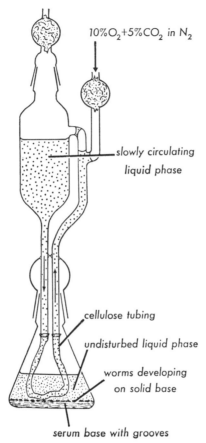

$10\%O_2 + 5\%CO_2$ in N_2

slowly circulating liquid phase

cellulose tubing

undisturbed liquid phase

worms developing on solid base

serum base with grooves

FIG. 78. A 'stationary' lift for *in vitro* cultivation of *Echinococcus granulosus*. Upper part based partly on Berntzen's recirculatory apparatus. By use of a cellulose tubing, the medium in the lower culture flask remains unagitated so that the interface between the worm and solid substrate is undisturbed; nutrients and waste materials can be exchanged via the cellulose membrane. (After Smyth & Miller, 1968.)

Other Cyclophyllidean Species

A number of early attempts to culture the larvae of various taeniid species have also been described; these generally failed to result in development.[406] A few more recent experiments with other species are now described.

Taenia crassiceps. Some partly successful experiments have been carried out with *T. crassiceps.* This is a useful experimental organism, as its larval stage undergoes vegetative reproduction in the peritoneal cavity of a mouse; moreover, it can be transferred by intraperitoneal injection. In Parker 199 and a gas phase of air $+5\%$ CO_2 in roller tubes, larvae underwent budding and developed scoleces.[330] Other complex media and gas phase of 10% $O_2 + 5\%$ CO_2 in N_2 has permitted survival of cysticerci with bud development for 1–4 months.[463] The continual flow technique used for other species (*Hymenolepis, Spirometra*) was not as successful as roller tubes with this species.[449]

Mesocestoides corti. Like *T. crassiceps,* this species has some potential for use as a laboratory organism as it can be maintained in mice by serial intraperitoneal passage. The adult worm is a parasite of carnivores; the first larval stage occurs in an oribatid mite and the second larval stage, which consists of a curiously branching *tetrathyridia,* occur in the body cavity and viscera of reptiles and mammals. It is relatively easy to culture tetrathyridia, which reproduce by asexual multiplication (by dividing or budding), in a variety of monophasic or diphasic media based on synthetic media such as M 115 or NCTC 109, supplemented with natural fluids.[439, 466]

Cultivation of Oncospheres to Metacestodes

Since cyclophyllid eggs can be obtained in very large numbers, from gravid proglottids, and readily hatched artificially (p. 122) it is surprising to find that few attempts have been made to grow oncospheres to metacestodes *in vitro.* Once hatching has been achieved, it is comparatively simple to prepare oncospheres in sterile culture by means of antibiotics. Oncospheres of *Taenia pisiformis* and *T. hydatigena* have been grown to large, actively moving vesicles in roller tubes, using Parker 858 with the appropriate host serum.[148, 148a]

Only two species, *Mesocestoides* sp.[464] and *H. nana*[28] have been grown to the infective metacestode stages *in vitro.* Oncospheres of *Mesocestoides* have been grown (in 8–12 weeks) axenically to small tetrathyridia which were infective to mice.[464] The culture medium consisted of NCTC 135 + 20–30% horse serum, used in stationary tubes at 30°C (gas phase not stated). *In vitro* development of *H. nana* oncospheres has been achieved in monoxenic culture.[28] Oncospheres were inoculated into rat fibroblast cultures, grown in NCTC 109 with

20% horse serum and a gas phase of 10% CO_2+30% O_2 in N_2. In four days these grew to cysticercoids, which were infective to rats. Since *H. nana* adults have been grown from cysticercoids *in vitro*[26] (p. 173), it can be said that the entire life cycle of this species has now been completed by Berntzen *in vitro*. The growth of the oncosphere of *H. nana* in axenic culture, however, has yet to be achieved.

11: Physiology of the Host-Parasite Relationship: I. Tissue Reactions

General Considerations

Host-parasite Interaction

With rare exceptions (e.g. *Hymenolepis nana*), a cestode makes contact with the tissues of at least two different hosts during its life-cycle. The degree of the response by each host to this contact is related to three main factors: (*a*) the nature of the tissue site invaded, (*b*) the intimacy of the host/parasite contact, and (*c*) the stage of development of the invading organism, i.e. whether adult or larva. For example, the host/parasite contacts established in the life-cycle of *Taenia saginata* are: (*a*) the scolex, when attached to the intestine in the definitive host, (*b*) the oncosphere, when penetrating the intestinal mucosa of the intermediate host and during its subsequent visceral migration and finally, (*c*) the developing larva in its final tissue site.

Before considering these host-parasite interactions in detail, some account of host ' defence ' mechanisms will be given. Nowadays, these mechanisms are generally discussed under the general (if slightly misleading) term ' immunity ', a term whose meaning is further discussed below. It is becoming increasingly important for the parasitologist to understand the basic principles of immunology, and an attempt is made here to summarise these briefly. Good general accounts are given in several texts.[175, 441]

Detailed consideration of immunological mechanisms as they apply to helminth parasites in vertebrates has been covered in several texts or reviews.[435, 436, 438, 441, 475, 479]

General Host Reactions

When a parasite (or other ' foreign ' i.e. ' non-self ' material; see p. 191) makes contact with a host at a cellular level, the host reacts by bringing into action types of ' defence ' measures which can broadly be grouped under two headings: (*a*) cellular (= tissue) reactions, (*b*) serological reactions. These overlap to some extent. In general, it can be said that a *tissue* reaction tends to be localised in the immediate site of the host-parasite contact; it may appear rapidly and often disappears after the invading material has left or has been destroyed. A *serological* effect (Chapter 12), on the other hand, is a more generalised effect, and one which may be considered to be a reaction of the whole body. These effects may sometimes, but not always, result in the establishment of 'immunity'. Theoretically, 'immunity' implies *freedom* from invasion by an organism; the term 'resistance' is also used in this context, although it implies that the defensive mechanisms of the host may not be completely successful in repelling the invasion of 'foreign' material. The terms 'immunity' and 'resistance' are, however, widely used as being synonymous and are generally so used in this text.

Vertebrate Cellular Reactions

The Inflammatory Reaction

The effect on tissues of the presence of a parasite is generally to invoke an *inflammatory* reaction, which plays an important role in the defence of the body against invasion of foreign tissue. It is thought that the host is able to distinguish between 'self' and 'non-self' material—the latter being defined as that which has a molecular configuration in some way different from that of the biological material normally present in the bloodstream or tissues of the host. There is no precise information, however, as to how this recognition is carried out at a molecular level. Recognition must occur on or near the surface of susceptible cells and probably it may require contact between the material and the recognising cell. The inflammatory process has been the subject of several reviews,[440, 442] and an excellent general account has been given by Sprent.[441]

If the amount of foreign material is small (e.g. an oncosphere) it may be gradually surrounded by phagocytic cells and immobilised by the deposition of collagenous tissue around it. If a large amount of foreign material (e.g. a cysticercus) is present, the reaction is much more severe; this is partly a result of mechanical irritation and partly the effect of released metabolic products on host cells.

The onset of inflammation is characterised by a local dilation of the capillaries (vasodilation). The latter is brought about by a number of factors of which a local nervous reaction and the release of a pharmacologically active agent, *histamine*, from specific cells termed *mast cells*, are probably the most important. Vasodilation results in an increase of blood supply to the affected area (= hyperemia) accompanied by an increased permeability of the capillary walls and the passage of protein materials from the blood into the tissue fluids. In the region of the invaded tissue, the vessel walls appear to become sticky, and poly-morphonuclear leucocytes (neutrophils) adhere to them. The leucocytes then proceed to infiltrate through the vessel walls and collect in large numbers at the site of invasion.

Leucocytes appear to be attracted by specific substances (e.g. leucotoxine) which may be released from damaged cells. Leucocyte infiltration is followed by lymphocytes, which are relatively undif-ferentiated cells whose function is obscure but some of them may become transformed into mononuclear cells or fibroblasts; the latter form the outer fibrous ' capsule ' which may surround metacestodes in certain tissue sites in intermediate hosts. In addition to histamine, other pharmacologically active substances—SRS-A (slow reacting substance), serotonin (5-hydroxytryptamine) and a polypeptide known as bradykinin—are released in tissues as a result of antigen-antibody reactions. The action of these substances in tissues is not fully understood.[175]

Cellular Reactions to Larval Cestodes

In mammalian intermediate hosts: general account. Most studies on tissue responses to metacestode infections have been carried out on those species of economic or medical importance which have a mammalian intermediate host, e.g. *Echinococcus* spp.;[275, 491] *Multiceps serialis*;[212] *Cysticercus cellulosae*;[399] *Cysticercus longicollis, T. crassiceps*;[107] *H. nana*.[20] There is also extensive literature on the patho-genesis of larval cestodes in fish,[21, 485] but little is known of the reactions in invertebrate hosts, such as insects or crustacea. An exception is the reaction of the flea, *Ctenocephalides felis*, to cysticercoids of *Dipylidium caninum* (p. 195).[63] In mammalian hosts (with a few exceptions) larval cestodes appear to be unusually immunogenic; and high, durable levels of acquired resistance to challenging infections may be stimulated by infection with even a few parasites. A further characteristic is the speed with which acquired immunity may develop, an effective level being reached, for example in the case of *H. nana* (p. 219) or *Hydatigera taeniaeformis* in rodents within one or two days.[475] This high immuno-genicity is likely to be related to the nature of the cestode tegument which, as stressed on p. 7, essentially consists of an ' exposed ' proto-plasmic surface which would permit the establishment of an exceedingly intimate contact between host and parasite.

It is not intended here to enter into a detailed description of the histopathological effects induced by metacestodes, but merely to give a generalised account of the pattern of response which occurs. It is important to note that not only does the degree of response vary from host to host, it varies (markedly in some species) with the 'strain' of a particular species of host and parasite and, furthermore, even in a single host the response may vary in different tissue sites. This has been clearly demonstrated in the case of *H. taeniaeformis*.[276] Thus, a strobilocercus developed to the infective stage in at least two strains of rats (Wistar, Gifu) and also in two strains of mouse (A, ARR). In other strains of mice, some development took place but thereafter degeneration occurred. There appears to be a gradation of the extent of the tissue reaction, extending from relatively slight in rats, more severe in the two 'suitable' mouse strains, and intense in the 'unsuitable' strains. In the suitable rat and mice strains, the slight tissue reaction was accompanied by the development of a cyst composed of connective tissue fibres within which the larvae could develop. In unsuitable hosts, accumulations of cells, mostly eosinophils, occurred around the parasite tissue, followed by a stratiform necrosis of granulation tissue. Eventually, the larva becomes necrotic and is overcome by granulation and sometimes calcification. Accumulation of histiocytes and the appearance of epithelioid cells and giant cells are also typical of this kind of reaction. The kind of response outlined above for *H. taeniaeformis* is typical of vertebrate tissue reactions, but its intensity can apparently vary even in the same site of a single host. For instance, in calves one cyst of *T. saginata* in muscle may survive, and yet an adjacent one may become necrotic. Such an effect may reflect nutritional, metabolic or immunological differences between sites—differences which may not become apparent without extremely detailed investigation.

The 'walling off' of an invading larva by an adventitious host capsule is common against cestodes, but in some cases the parasite also secretes a covering layer. This is the case with the developing cyst of the hydatid organism, *Echinococcus granulosus*, which secretes a PAS-positive layer around itself, even during *in vitro* culture. The layers of the cyst wall which are finally formed are, however, complex (p. 180) and their origins are difficult to determine precisely.

Reactions to larval Hymenolepis nana. Although this species has been widely used as an experimental model in studies on cestode immunity its histopathology has not been extensively studied. The importance of this species is the fact that it can either complete its entire life cycle in the same host or utilise an intermediate host (Fig. 1). In the former case, fed oncospheres hatch in the intestine and rapidly penetrate the villi to develop to cysticercoids. No cellular infiltration occurs until about 72 hours;[20] and at 96 hours, when cysticercoids are fully developed, cellular infiltration becomes marked, eosinophils and lymphocytes being especially involved.   Fibrocytes do not appear, nor, it seems is a capsule formed around the parasite within a villus (Fig. 79).   When mice infected with cysticercoids are challenged with oncospheres (p. 219), almost none (Table 40) penetrate the mucosa;   and

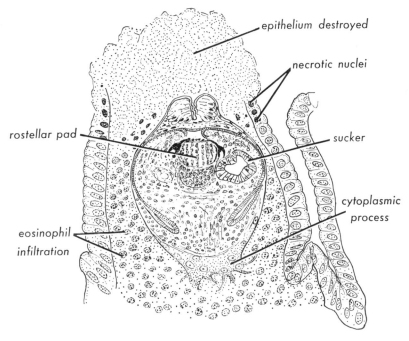

FIG. 79. Section of a cysticercoid of *Hymenolepis nana* in an intestinal villus of the mouse; 96 hours post-infection.   No fibrous host capsule is formed but marked eosinophilia develops.   (Original.)

those which do, induce an inflammatory reaction earlier than in a previously uninfected mouse.   Blood eosinophilia is also associated with *H. nana* in mice.[18]   As shown in Fig. 80, a high level of eosinophilia develops during the first 20 days, to be followed by a latent period, followed in time by a second increase at 80–90 days—the latter presumably being due to reinfection by eggs released from worms matured after the initial infection.[18]   It is also well known that infections of parasitic worms not only induce an increased mast cell secretion, but also stimulate mitosis of partially degranulated mast cells, with an increase in mast cell number.[104]   The increase of mast cells in mice naturally infected with *H. nana* and the nematode *Syphacia* (Fig. 81) is, however, much less than that which occurs in mice infected with *Schistosoma*.

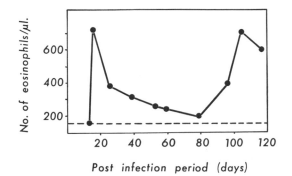

FIG. 80. Blood eosinophilia related to the presence of *Hymenolepis nana* in mice. (After Bailenger, *et al.*, 1961.)

In invertebrate hosts. The tissue reactions of invertebrates to parasite invasion have been very little studied in relation to cestodes, although more information is available regarding trematode and arthropod parasites.[173, 355, 422] The general reaction of invertebrates

TABLE 40

Induction of resistance of Hymenolepis nana *by previous infection. Mice initially infected with* 18 500 *eggs and challenged with* 21 300 *eggs on the tenth day*

(Data modified from Bailey[20])

	Experimental Animals			Control Animals (challenge infection only)		
Mouse no.	Hrs. after infection	Total no. of larvae		Mouse no.	Hrs. after infection	Total no. of larvae
T-15	18	0		T-21	96	51
T-16	48	0				
T-17	72	0				

to cestode larva is to attempt to encapsulate the parasite by means of a haemocytic reaction. Thus, the cysticercoids of *Anomotaenia pyriformis* become encapsulated in the coelom of the earthworm *Lumbriculus variegatus*,[355] and the cysticercoids of *D. caninum* become encapsulated in the cat flea, *Ctenocephalides felis*.

A detailed account of the latter process has been given;[63] briefly, it occurs as follows: The blood of fleas contains three types of haemocytes: preamoebocytes, amoebocytes and macrocytes; and all appear to be involved in the response to infections of cestode larva.   The haemocyte response appears to be slow, and no increase in the number takes place until the fifth day of infection. This results in an aggregation of haemocytes, chiefly amoebocytes, in which a cysticercoid may become embedded. A capsule two or three layers thick forms around a cysticercoid and the encapsulated larva may die and become transformed into a mass of yellow pigment.   During the pupal stage, haemocytes which have not already formed a capsule around the parasites apparently disregard the cestode tissue and carry on their normal function, namely to dissolve the larval host tissues.

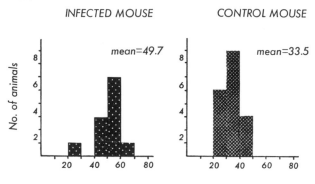

INFECTED MOUSE   CONTROL MOUSE

No. of Mast cells/mm² skin

FIG. 81. Increase in mast cells in skin of mice infected
with *Hymenolepis nana* and *Syphacia* (nematode). (After
Fernex & Fernex, 1962.)

It is well known that larvae of pseudophyllidean cestodes also produce pathogenic effects in fish.[485]   Effects due to various genera of Diphyllobothriiidae, especially *Diphyllobothrium*, *Ligula* and *Schisto-cephalus*, have been described.   *Diphyllobothrium* plerocercoids can occur in almost any tissue, such as muscle or liver, or lie free in the body cavity.   The host tissue capsule may, however, be so thin and so closely applied to the worm tissue that it appears to be part of it.   The same situation occurs with the large progenetic plerocercoids of *Schisto-cephalus solidus*, which apparently lie free in the body cavity;   histo-logical examination reveals, however, that larvae are covered in a thin non-cellular layer which may be of host origin.   The marked patho-genesis of *Diphyllobothrium* larvae is probably related to a seasonal rise in temperature, which stimulates plerocercoids to burst out of their tissue site and migrate through other tissues.

In addition to the normal tissue reactions, heavy infections of large plerocercoids, such as *Ligula*, can induce parasitic castration in the roach, *Leuciscus rutilus*.   This effect is associated with the cytological changes in the basophil cells of the middle glandular region of the pituitary and a reduction in the secretion of gonadotrophic hormones;[197, 485] in fish infected with *Ligula* a marked increase in the number of polymorphonuclear leucocytes and monocytes in the blood has been reported.[485] The effects produced by plerocercoids of *Schistocephalus* are not so marked as with *Ligula*; gonad maturation is retarded but not stopped, although the normal spawning behaviour of the fish host is disrupted.[15]

Induction of sarcoma by cestode tissue. The strobilocercus of *Hydatigera taeniaeformis* is unusual in that it induces hepatic sarcoma in the rat liver—malignant tumours arising from infections of more than 250 days' duration.[372] The tumours appear to rise from the fibrous capsule formed by the host around the larva and not from the liver tissue itself. The active agent inducing these sarcomas has not been identified, but multiple peritoneal sarcomas have been obtained by injecting rats with suspensions of washed, ground *Hydatigera* larvae obtained from rats of the same strain which were susceptible to cysticercus-induced sarcoma.[96] The sera of infected rats has also been examined electrophoretically. It is interesting to note that rats of a different strain did not develop tumours when similarly injected. Larvae 6–10 months old produced inactive suspensions, but carcinogenic activity was present in 12-month old larvae. The induction of sarcoma by this organism is clearly a field which calls for further study.

Cellular Reactions to Adult Cestodes

A useful review on the pathogenesis of adult cestodes has been made by Rees.[322] The closeness of the attachment of the scolex to the gut (Chapter 3) is clearly important in relation to pathogenesis. It is not possible to generalise about the cellular reactions developed. Many species, perhaps a majority, invoke no reactions; others may produce inflammation, eosinophilia or fibrosis in association with hyperplasia or metaplasia. Occasionally, necrotic nodules or abscesses may develop.

The lack of cellular response in the gut may prove to be typical of many cestodes and may be related to the rapid turnover of the mucosal cells, a situation which would give little time for a response to develop. For example, in the gut of a dog, *Echinococcus* evokes no marked cellular reaction, even though the scolex enters and dilates the crypts of Lieberkühn and invades the lamina propria in some instances. (Figs. 12, 73). However, antibodies may be detected in canine serum, and the latter gives a strong serological reaction with adult worms (p. 210, Figs. 85, 86). Adult *H. nana* similarly provokes little tissue reaction in the mouse gut (Fig. 6).

A few examples of species pathogenic in the adult stage are quoted below; for a comprehensive summary see Rees.[322]   In the Pseudo-phyllidea, the scolex generally does little damage.   An exception is *Parabothrium gadi-pollachii* and *Abothrium gadi* which causes extreme fibrosis in the mucosa of *Gadus* spp.[482]   *Raillietina echinobothrida* may also be pathogenic in birds.[322]

In the Tetraphyllidea, although species armed with hooks tear the mucosa, no inflammatory reaction results.[322]   In birds, the mucosa may be extensively damaged by the adult scolex of cyclophyllids.   Thus, the scoleces of the *Hymenolepis parvula* and *Aploparaxis furcigera* induce a chronic inflammation in the mucosa of duck,[398] with massive invasion of eosinophils and plasma cells into the infected area.   In these cases (especially in *A. furugera*) the size of the scolex is such that it dilates the crypt walls, eventually damaging them sufficiently to cause bleeding.

12: Physiology of the Host-Parasite Relationship: II. Antigen-Antibody Reactions

Basic Concepts of Immunology

Antigens and Antibodies

In addition to the tissue reactions described in the previous chapter, the invasion of a vertebrate host by ' foreign ' material is associated with a number of serological (or humoral) reactions, so-called because they are manifested particularly by the serum of an infected host. Material which invokes these reactions is said to be *antigenic* and the molecules it releases or exposes to the host are termed *antigens*.

Antigens are macromolecules of protein or complex polysaccharides (but see *haptens*, below). In order to act as an antigen, a molecule must generally have a minimal molecular weight of about 10 000 and a surface configuration of certain chemical groups. For a chemical grouping to be ' foreign ', it need only present a configuration which is unfamiliar to the organism, and the extent of the host response is apparently determined by the extent of the ' foreignness ' of the antigen. The antigenicity of proteins is determined by both their structure and the nature of their chemical groupings. Lipids are not directly antigenic but may act as *haptens*—substances which, when coupled to proteins or complex polysaccharides can dictate specificity of the coupled ' antigen '.

Helminth antigens are sometimes classified either as *somatic* or as *metabolic* antigens, but it is not yet possible to say how far this distinction can be justified. *Somatic* antigens—also known as *endogenous* or *structural* antigens[479]—are believed to be molecules attached to, or released from, the exposed surface of a parasite body, such as the tegument. *Metabolic*—also known as *exogenous* antigens or *exoantigens*— are defined as being metabolic products, such as excretory or secretory materials, which are released by the parasite during growth, development or tissue penetration.

The introduction of antigen provokes the appearance in the blood and tissue fluids of a soluble protein entity termed *antibody* which has the property of combining with its specific antigen.

It is usual to classify plasma proteins, on the basis of separation by electrophoresis, into four groups, namely albumin and α-, β- and γ-globulins. It was formerly thought that antibodies occurred either in the γ-globulins or (especially in ungulates) in the β-globulins. This generalisation, however, has proved to be an over-simplification, for some antibody has been detected with a component lying between the γ and β-globulins; this is sometimes termed T-globulin or γ_1-globulin. High-speed centrifugation methods have also been used to separate plasma proteins and on the basis of their sedimentation constants (Svedberg units) fractions termed 7S γ-globulin and 19S macroglobulin have been identified. Since the 7S fraction can be further subdivided, it is clear that definition of γ-globulin solely in terms of electrophoretic mobility can no longer be accepted, and the general term *immunoglobulins* is now used to describe the group of closely related proteins involved in antibody activity.

The mechanism whereby antibodies are produced is still a matter of controversy, although the 'clonal selection theory' of Burnet[175] appears, at present, to be the hypothesis most generally accepted.

Antigen-Antibody Interactions

When antibodies react against antigens they may combine with them and form precipitates or they may cause clumping of cells (such as foreign blood cells) which bear antigenic surfaces, or they may provoke a number of other reactions—such as lysis; these reactions are discussed below.

In vitro, the proportions in which antigens and antibodies are present has a marked effect on the degree of precipitation taking place. Thus, maximum precipitation occurs when the amount of antigen is equivalent to (Fig. 82), or just in excess of, the amount of antibody. With extreme excess of antigen or antibody, precipitation is greatly reduced or may not occur at all. Antigen-antibody reactions are also complicated by the fact that some antibody may occur in a 'non-precipitating' form; such antibodies are monovalent, i.e. with one combining site.

Serum, obtained from an animal invaded by a particular parasite and containing antibodies to it, is termed *antiserum* (or sometimes, perhaps less aptly, *immune* serum), and the resulting type of immunity conferred on the host is termed *active immunity*. Immunity can also be transferred into a non-immune host by injection of antiserum, and immunity induced in this way is termed *passive* immunity, since the recipient animal has not itself taken part in the establishment of the immune state. In contrast with active immunity, passive immunity is usually short-lasting.

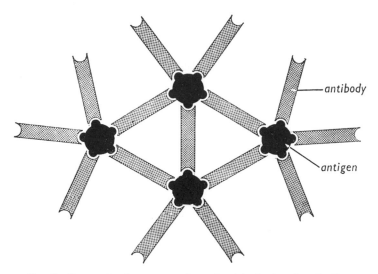

FIG. 82. Interaction between antigens (multivalent) and antibodies (bivalent). (After Smyth, 1962b.)

Serological Tests for Antigen or Antibody

General account. Antibody concentration is expressed as the *titre* of a serum sample. This is the reciprocal of the highest dilution of serum giving a detectable reaction; it is expressed as the number of (arbitrary) antibody units per unit volume of undiluted serum. Although this nomenclature is widely used, it has the disadvantage of not measuring antibody in absolute weight units. The technical details of methods for measuring titres are beyond the scope of this book, but are dealt with in laboratory manuals.[50, 478]

Routine tests. Some methods commonly used in serology are outlined below:

Precipitation. When suitable concentrations of antigen and antibody are mixed *in vitro*, the solution becomes turbid and insoluble antigen-antibody complex precipitates out.

Agglutination. This phenomenon is essentially the same as that of precipitation, except that the antigens brought together by antibodies are either particulate or cellular (e.g. bacteria, yeasts, erythrocytes).   Agglutination of red blood cells is referred to by a special term, *haemagglutination.*

The range and sensitivity of the haemagglutination reaction have been considerably extended by the observation that erythrocytes, after treatment with tannic acid (a mordant), can absorb many protein antigens at their surface; polysaccharides can be absorbed without tannic acid treatment.   Other particles—such as polystyrene, latex, collodion, sephadex or bentonite—can similarly be coated with antigens and hence used as ' carriers '.   Particles or cells treated in this way are exceedingly sensitive and can detect as little as 0·003 μgm of antibody (measured as nitrogen).

Complement fixation.   This is a phenomenon related to the properties of a component of serum termed ' complement '.   Complement was discovered when it was shown that fresh serum lost some of its cytotoxic activity when heated to 56°C and kept at that temperature for 30 minutes.   Complement appears to be a substance made up of at least six factors or components which act in a definitive sequence to damage certain cells; its physical nature is not understood.   Complement is present in greatly varying proportions in sera of different animals, but the level is constant for each species.   Guinea-pig serum contains more complement than most other sera and is widely used in experimental work.

When antigen and antibody react to form an antigen-antibody complex in serum, complement becomes actually bound up (= absorbed) in the complex, and hence removed from the serum.   This process is termed ' complement fixation '.   This reaction of complement with the antigen-antibody complex can be used to detect the presence of a specific antigen or antibody; but, since this reaction occurs without causing any observable effect, a haemolytic system must be used to make the effect visible.   Normally, sensitised sheep erythrocytes (see below) are used, as these will lyse when added to complement, thus:

(sheep   erythrocytes+antibody)+complement————→   haemolysis

but, if the complement has been bound by another antigen-antibody complex, haemolysis will not take place.

In a complement-fixation test (Fig. 83), serum (heated to inactivate its own complement), suspected of containing antibodies to a particular parasite, is mixed with standard parasite antigen and added to fresh guinea-pig serum (as complement source).   ' Sensitised ' sheep erythrocytes (i.e. those mixed with (heated) antiserum prepared against them in a rabbit) are added and, if the cells lyse, the levels of free complement has remained high and the serum is negative for parasite antibody

(Fig. 83).   On the other hand, if no haemolysis occurs, the complement has been bound by the parasite antigen-antibody complex and the test serum is positive for antibodies to the parasite.

Hypersensitivity and intradermal reactions.   Hypersensitivity is a peculiar reaction characterised by a heightened response to invasion by foreign substances.   For instance, when a guinea-pig is injected with

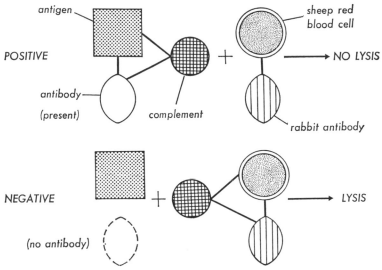

Fig. 83. The complement-fixation reaction.   (Adapted from Humphrey & White, 1964.)

a small quantity of foreign protein (e.g. a milligram of ovalbumin) it becomes 'sensitised' to that protein.   If a further challenging dose (one milligram) of antigen is given, two or three weeks later, the body suffers a violent general systemic reaction (anaphylaxis) which results in death within a few minutes.

Hypersensitivity is due, partly to the effect of a special type of antibody, termed a *reaginic* antibody, and partly to the release of pharmacologically active substances—notably histamine, serotonin (5-hydroxytryptamine), SRS-A (slow reacting substance), and bradykinin.   The source of histamine is the mast cell (p. 191).   By restriction of the antigen to a small area of skin, local hypersensitivity may be produced.   These intradermal reactions are useful in the diagnosis of certain diseases of helminth origin (e.g. hydatidiasis, p. 213), the test being carried out by injecting an extract of the parasite or placing some powdered parasite on a small area of previously scarified skin.

A positive result is indicated if a weal develops in the test area within 10–20 minutes. A useful review of the effects of antigen-antibody complexes in living systems, with particular reference to helminth infections, has been made by W.H.O.[479]

Detection of Antigens and Antibodies

Immunodiffusion

General principles. Under appropriate conditions, antigens and antibodies combine to form insoluble precipitates (p. 200), and extensive use has been made of this phenomenon to develop sensitive methods for the detection of these substances. Most methods involve the use of gels, such as agar or other support media, the general principle of the method being termed *immunodiffusion*. Elegant methods of ever increasing discrimination are now available, and are dealt with in practical texts;[50, 85, 478] application of the method to helminth material, in particular, has been reviewed by Kent.[194, 195]

In immunodiffusion techniques, antigen and antibody are allowed to diffuse towards each other in agar and one or more precipitation bands are formed, according to the number of specific reactants present, i.e. a complex mixture of antigens will produce a number of bands (Fig. 84).

Double diffusion in tubes. The antibody and antigen are each most conveniently mixed with agar and separated by a layer of pure agar. Precipitation bands form in the middle layer and, with strong antisera, may appear within a couple of hours (Fig. 84A). Although this method is very sensitive and can detect 0·3–0·9 μgm of antibody nitrogen, it has its limitations. Thus, the number of bands observed in agar tubes does not necessarily indicate the total number of antigen-antibody systems present, because in complex mixtures some of the bands may be hidden by others. Such complex mixtures can be identified only by procedures of high resolving power, such as immuno-electrophoresis (p. 205).

Double diffusion in plates. Various modifications of techniques involving diffusion in plates are widely used for parasite antigens which have complex systems. They are especially valuable in comparing two antigens with reference to one antiserum and *vice versa*. The technique depends on the diffusion of antigen and antibody towards each other from troughs or wells cut in agar. Such plates are known as Ouchterlony plates, after the inventor. If antigen and antibody are simultaneously allowed to diffuse from such troughs at right angles, a narrow line of precipitate is formed (Fig. 84B). If it is required to examine more than one antigen or antibody, a series of cups can be cut out and the lines of precipitation compared (Figs. 84C, 84D). Antibodies can also be labelled with dyes or isotopes to increase still further the sensitivity of the methods.

Immuno-electrophoresis. This technique consists of the electrophoretic separation of a mixture of antigens carried out on a supporting

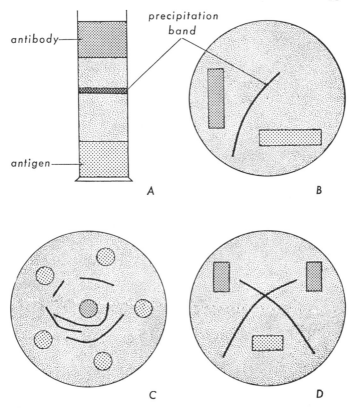

FIG. 84. Various forms of double diffusion-in-gel techniques. A, Tube technique of Oudin. B, C, D, Variations of the plate technique of Ouchterlony. (After Smyth, 1966.)

medium such as agar, gelatin or cellulose acetate paper. This is followed by the linear application of antiserum, which is allowed to diffuse towards the separated components (Fig. 87). Conversely the antiserum may be separated by electrophoresis and the antigen applied linearly.

Fluorescent Antibody Techniques

These make use of the fact that proteins may be labelled with fluorescent dyes, such as fluorescein isothiocyanate or rhodamine B.

These dyes have the property of absorbing ultra-violet light between 290-495 mμ and emitting a longer wavelength (525 mμ) green light. Thus, the protein labelled with the dye can be visualised by fluorescent microscopy. The method is particularly valuable for the precise localisation of an antigen in or on a parasite; the immunological identity of the mucopolysaccharide covering *Echinococcus* protoscoleces (p. 180) has been identified by this procedure. It has also been used with *Hymenolepis*.[78, 80] The method has the disadvantage that the absorbed fluorochrome is rapidly 'burnt' out in ultraviolet light so that the observation time is very limited.

Serological Reactions in Specific Cestode Infections

General Account

For the most part, serological reactions in cestode infections have been confined to the Diphyllobothriidae among the Pseudophyllidea and the Taeniidae among the Cyclophyllidea. Most of the main methods of assaying antibody, described above, have been used in helminth infections. Those chiefly used include:

(a) *in vitro* reactions with living material, (b) electrophoresis of serum, (c) immunodiffusion techniques, and (d) immuno-electrophoresis.

In vitro *Reactions with Living Cestode Material*

In the case of nematode and trematode infections, a strong antibody titre frequently develops, and when adults or larvae are placed in antiserum from an infected host they become covered in a surface precipitate of an antigen-antibody complex. The best known reaction is perhaps the *Cercarienhüllenreaktion*, in which an envelope develops around schistosome cercariae.[422]

Curiously enough, little similar work has been carried out with living cestode material, a result undoubtedly due to the fact that, whereas many larval stages of trematodes and nematodes are free-living and easily obtained, most cestode larval stages are parasitic (except coracidia) and much more difficult to handle *in vitro*. It is possible that some serological reactions with living cestodes have been overlooked owing to their nature not being recognised by observers.

(a) *Oncosphere.* One of the earliest serological reactions in cestodes was described by Silverman,[388] who showed that calf and rabbit antisera, from calves and rabbits infected with the cysticerci, gave reactions with the hatched and activated oncospheres of *T. saginata* and *T. pisiformis* respectively. Three types of reactions were noted:

(i) the formation of precipitates around the secretions of the penetrating glands and at other points on the embryos, (ii) the formation of a membrane enclosing the entire embryo and its secretions, and (iii) a lethal and lytic effect.

It is important to stress that these reactions were obtained with *hatched* oncospheres which had been activated in an enzyme-bile solution (Table 33), for without this treatment the oncosphere remains protected by the oncospheral membrane. This may account for the fact that rat antiserum has been reported as giving no reactions against the hatched but inactivated hexacanth embryos of *H. taeniaeformis*.[64] The lethal and lytic effect noted above was observed in control (i.e. normal) serum so that many normal sera may similarly contain agents lytic to the oncospheres. These results further indicate that cysticerci and oncospheres of *T. pisiformis* and *T. saginata* must share antigens, a phenomenon well known from other helminths.

TABLE 41

Infectivity of eggs of Hymenolepis nana *in white mice after 24 hours incubation in anti-adult* (Hymenolepis) *rabbit antiserum or in normal rabbit serum*

(Data from Heyneman & Welsh[156])

Serum lot	% infection in eggs after incubation	
	in antiserum	in normal serum
1	0·2	3·9
2	0·2	4·1
3	0·2	3·9
4	0·3	3·5
5	0·1	3·6
average	0·2	3·8

That adult cestodes can also have antigens in common with both eggs and cysticercoids (see below) has been shown for *H. nana*.[156] When homogenised adult worms of this species were injected into rabbits, the antisera produced gave reactions with eggs, cysticercoids and adults. Reactions noted with one-third of the eggs were: (i) retraction of central egg membrane away from the embryophore, (ii) appearance of a granular precipitate within the eggs near the outer wall, and (iii) agglutination of eggs into groups of 2–10. Up to 10% of eggs in normal serum showed somewhat similar reactions. Eggs incubated in immune serum also showed greatly reduced infectivity to white mice (Table 41).

(b) *Larval cestodes.* When homogenates or extracts of cestode tissue, whether adult or larval, are injected into rabbits, they will induce the corresponding antibodies. If living cestode tissue of the same species is now placed in this antiserum it can be expected that antibody-antigen reactions such as precipitation, will occur at the surface of the live worms. This is borne out by the limited experimental work carried out. Thus, cysticercoids of *H. nana* in anti-adult rabbit antiserum show a characteristic cuticular bubbling, and the rostellum and sucker activity is affected; normal rabbit serum also produces a slight effect.[156] In the natural host, however, the level of antibodies evoked is low, and cysticercoids show no reaction in antiserum from a mouse infection.

As with *H. nana*, when protoscoleces of *Echinococcus* are placed in anti-protoscolex rabbit or guinea-pig antiserum, the scolex evaginates and precipitates occur around the rostellum and the tegument, and at the excretory pores.[383] Protoscoleces were found to give the same reaction in serum of humans suffering from hydatid disease—even apparently in cases of many years duration.[383] This reaction can therefore be used as a serological test for hydatid disease in man. In *in vitro* culture, protoscoleces show a tendency to aggregate by their posterior bladders[429] (p. 179), an effect related to the appearance of a sticky PAS-positive layer (p. 180)—which may prove in part to be an antigen-antibody precipitate—in this region (Fig. 85B).

A number of interesting serological reactions have also been observed with the plerocercoids of pseudophyllidean cestodes. It has been found that sera from a large number of fish species are lethal to plerocercoids of *Spirometra mansonoides*, precipitates being formed on the tegument, as in mouse sera (Plate IV, Fig. A). Fish extracts also reacted *in vitro*.[256] Sera from other species proved to be non-toxic and presumably these species could act as potential hosts.

The exact kind of immunological mechanism involved in these reactions has not been determined. In the natural mouse host, it can be demonstrated that antibodies to *Spirometra mansonoides* are developed. Normal mouse serum produced some precipitation with the sparganum on the scolex; whereas spargana placed in immune serum from an infected mouse produced a flocculent precipitate around the body of the worms within six hours.[258] This precipitate (Plate IV, Fig. A) differs from that which forms on the scolex in normal serum or in culture media containing serum. The latter probably represents a non-antibody (?) reaction with a secretion from glands in this region—an effect somewhat similar to that described for the scolex of *Echinococcus* (Plate IV, Fig. D) and the penetration glands of oncospheres (p. 207).

Adult cestodes. Relatively few studies of the serological reactions of adult cestodes *in vitro* have been made. It has been stressed (p. 197) that, since adult cestodes are intestinal parasites, the immunological response is generally small, except where severe destruction of the host intestinal epithelium occurs. 'Immune' sera from infected hosts will, therefore, generally possess only low levels of antibody. This

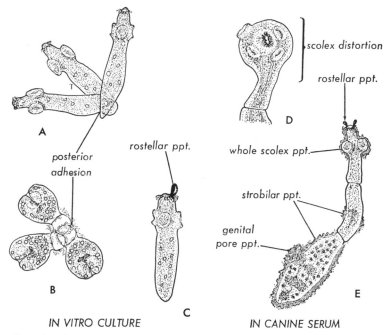

IN VITRO CULTURE   IN CANINE SERUM

FIG. 85. Some serological reactions with *Echinococcus*. A. Strobilar agglutination in culture. B. 'Posterior bladder' agglutination in culture. C. Antigen-antibody reaction with rostellar gland secretion in culture. D. Scolex distortion in canine antiserum. E. Tegumental reaction in canine antiserum. (Original.)

conclusion is on the whole borne out by the few experiments carried out. Thus, although young adult *H. nana* will form a precipitate with anti-adult rabbit serum,[156] it gives no directly observable reactions with 'immune' serum from a normal mouse host.[475] However, by use of immunofluorescent staining, it can be shown that antibodies combine with adult worms *in situ*;[78, 80] some of the stimulating exoantigens appear to be esterases.[81]

Antibody to *H. nana* has been detected in intestinal mucus, even in uninfected mice.[475] After three hours in normal mucosal extract some

5% of worms died, others showed muscular inactivity, but some 80% were active. In contrast, in 'immune' mucosal extract, activity generally ceased in most worms and after four hours incubation, a distinct membrane—somewhat reminiscent of the *Cercarienhüllen-reaktion* of trematodes[422]—appeared around some of the worms. Adult *Echinococcus* may prove to be more sensitive to antibody-antigen reactions than protoscoleces and a number of serological reactions have been observed.[429] The most reactive region appears to be the rostellum and the secretion from this reacts with hydatid fluid, bovine, canine or horse serum (Fig. 85). The material reacting with the scolex secretion may be a 'natural' antibody. During *in vitro* culture (p. 183)

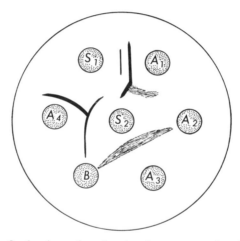

Fig. 86. Ouchterlony plate showing the presence of antibodies to *Echinococcus granulosus* in the sera of infected animals. $S_1 =$ canine serum 33 days after oral infection with *E. granulosus* protoscoleces. $S_2 =$ mouse serum 150 days after intraperitoneal inoculation of protoscoleces of *E. granulosus*. $A_1 = E.$ *granulosus* from the dog 33 days after ingestion of protoscoleces. $A_2 = E.$ *granulosus* from the dog 21 days after ingestion of protoscoleces. $A_3 =$ protoscoleces of *E. granulosus* from the sheep. $A_4 =$ sheep hydatid fluid concentrated 10X by ammonium sulphate precipitation. B = Blank well (Control). (After Smith & Smyth, 1968.)

in media containing hydatid fluid, a marked scolex secretion develops in some specimens (Plate IV, Fig. D), and remains attached to the rostellum. Since hydatid fluid contains some antibody[402a] this may be a true antigen-antibody precipitate. Immune canine serum from a 33-day old infection, has been shown to contain antibody to adult *Echinococcus*[402a] (Fig. 86). In such serum a vigorous reaction was observed with live worms *in vitro* (Table 42 and Fig. 85); a precipitate appeared around the terminal proglottid, and the scolex invaginated and became distorted. This may partly represent a complement-boosted reaction, for in inactivated serum from the same source it did not occur. Other types of precipitation that may cause aggregation (Fig. 85) have been observed *in vitro*, and a complex antigen pattern appears to occur in adult *Echinococcus*.[402a, 429]

Electrophoresis of Sera

Electrophoresis of sera as a means of detecting serological differences has now been largely replaced by immunodiffusion and immuno-electrophoresis (see below). Early work with *Cysticercus fasciolaris* showed that a qualitative difference existed between the sera of normal and infected rats.[206]

Immunodiffusion

General account. Within recent years, this technique has been extensively used to detect and identify helminth antigens and host antibodies. Only a few examples of the many species studied will be considered here, but the introduction of these methods has virtually revolutionised isolation and identification of helminth antigens. Early precipitation techniques indicated that the extract of a particular cestode appeared to contain only a small number of antigens, but immunodiffusion techniques have generally shown that, in fact, many more antigens are present. Application of immuno-electrophoresis techniques has enabled even further separation of antigens to be made, and the separation of antigens of *Echinococcus* is treated in detail below. One of the interesting results which these techniques have revealed has been that helminths from different phyla, such as nematodes and trematodes, share antigens with cestodes. Thus, *T. saginata* has been shown to share antigens with the trematodes *Fasciola hepatica*, *Schistosoma mansoni*, *Dicrocoelium dendriticum* and the nematode *Onchocerca volvulus*.[31] A more expected result is that different species or genera of cestodes also share antigens. Thus, *Diphyllobothrium mansoni* and *Moniezia* sp., share antigens,[140] as do several species of Taeniidae.[113–116] Some of the antigens of different species appear to be identical; for example, electrophoresis could reveal no difference between the water-soluble antigens of *M. expansa* and *M. benedeni*.[265]

Analysis of cestode antigens is inevitably related to their protein and polysaccharide composition, and a number of the more common species have been investigated. For example, chemical fractionation[235] of *T. saginata* has revealed the presence of five protein (nucleoprotein) and three polysaccharide fractions, although it is likely that the number

TABLE 42

Serological reactions of adult Echinococcus granulosus *with various sera. Adult worms were removed from a dog and cultured in Medium 199 + 20% α γ calf serum before testing* (NR = no reaction.) (Data from Smyth & Miller[429])

| Exposure time (hrs.) | Control: α γ calf serum | Infected dog serum | | Test Media (37°C.) | | |
		normal	inactivated*	Normal bovine serum	Normal horse serum	Hydatid fluid
0·5	NR	ppt. terminal proglottid	NR	scolex secretion	scolex secretion	scolex secretion
1	NR	rostellar invagination	scolex secretion	no change	no change	no change
2	NR	dark and contracted	no change	no change	no change	no change
11	scolex secretion	degenerating	no change : v. active	post proglottids sticky	no change	no change
24	no change : v. active	just surviving	no change : v. active	no change : v. active	no change : v. active	becoming darker?

* 30 mins. at 56°C.

of antigens isolated by sensitive methods may be much greater than can be detected by chemical methods.

Antigens in Echinococcus. Analysis of the antigens in this species can serve as a useful example of how cestode antigens are studied. On account of its relatively great medical interest and the importance of establishing sensitive and accurate methods of diagnosing hydatid disease, the antigens of *Echinococcus* have been intensively studied.[421] Nearly all the work on *Echinococcus* antigens have been concerned with the larval (i.e. hydatid) stage and crude hydatid fluid, filtered or

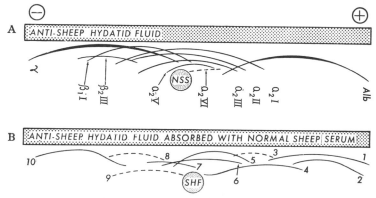

FIG. 87. Identification of parasite and host antigens in hydatid fluid (19 antigenic components) by immuno-electrophoresis. A. normal sheep serum (NSS) against anti-sheep hydatid fluid (from rabbit). The lines represent the 9 *host* antigens. B. Sheep hydatid fluid (SHF) against anti-sheep hydatid fluid (from rabbit) after absorption with NSS: only the 10 parasite components remain (see p. 214). (After Chordi & Kagan, 1965.)

unfiltered extracts of protoscoleces, or cyst walls or fractions of these have been used as antigens; but the procedures whereby their antigens have been obtained and utilised by different workers have varied considerably. These antigens have been used for the diagnosis of hydatid disease by a number of different serological procedures, of which the Casoni skin reaction, the complement fixation test, the bentonite flocculation test and the indirect haemagglutination tests are the best known.[421] Although false positives can be obtained in some of these tests (i.e. positives due to various collagen diseases) the careful and critical use of these tests can be valuable for diagnostic purposes.[186]

An example of how techniques for antigen analysis have improved is seen in the study of hydatid fluid. Early work[66] detected nine components in hydatid fluid by analysing anti-hydatid fluid (A-HF) antisera produced in rabbits.[66] Later work with immuno-electrophoresis and Ouchterlony plates detected no fewer than nineteen and twenty-three antigens respectively.[66] The main antigens were identified by the former method, but the latter method detected the very weak antigens also. Of the nineteen strong antigenic components, nine were of host origin and ten of parasite origin. This conclusion is clear from Fig. 87.A in which normal sheep serum (NSS) has been run against anti-sheep hydatid fluid, i.e. anti-sera developed (in rabbits) as a result of injections of sheep hydatid fluid. The reaction clearly results in nine bands, which indicates that the hydatid fluid contained nine antigens which had originated from host serum. Similarly, in Fig. 87.B sheep hydatid fluid (SHF) is run against the same anti-sheep hydatid fluid (from rabbits) which, this time, has been absorbed with normal sheep serum, so that the host antigens have been precipitated and removed. The ten bands which appear are thus clearly of parasite origin.

Various modifications of this kind of approach will undoubtedly lead to clarification and identification of the antigens of many species of cestodes.

13 : Physiology of the Host-Parasite Relationship : III. Immunological Reactions to Cestodes : Innate and Acquired Resistance

Innate Resistance

General Considerations

The mechanisms which prevent the establishment of a parasite within a particular host vary so widely from species to species that they are impossible to define in general terms. If, through suitable ecological conditions, a parasite makes contact with a potential host and yet fails to become established in it, the host is said to possess *innate* or *natural* resistance (or immunity) to that parasite. Several reviews of this field are available.[211, 381] Although the word ' resistance ' —which implies that an active process of defence (in a ' military sense ') is taking place—is widely used, in many instances an alternative term, *insusceptibility*, would be more appropriate. Insusceptibility implies that adverse anatomical, behavioural, ecological, or physiological features of the host eliminate the possibility of a parasite becoming established in that particular host. Thus, a copepod may be insusceptible to invasion by a pseudophyllid larva because of the thickness of its gut wall. Again, as was discussed earlier (p. 24), the physiological conditions in a particular vertebrate gut—with regard to pH, pCO_2, pO_2, E_h or some other physico-chemical characteristic— may be such that it provides an unfavourable site in relation to the metabolism of a particular species. It has also been shown that the sera of some animals have ' natural ' antibodies which react with a parasite, although the host may not previously have come in contact with such a parasite (p. 208). Again, the diet of the host, which can have a profound effect on the growth rate of cestodes, may be lacking in a nutritional factor essential for the parasite's development. Some of these factors may change with age, so that an 'age resistance' occurs with some species.   The terms 'insusceptibility', 'resistance' and 'immunity', thus clearly overlap and are not capable of definition in precise terms.   The whole problem of resistance is further complicated by the occurrence of strains of both host and parasite; and genetic considerations must, therefore, also be taken into account (p. 5).

A resistance which is *innate* must be distinguished from one which is *acquired* as a result of a previous invasion of a parasite.   The latter is considered below.

Acquired Resistance (Immunity)

General Considerations

It has been seen (Chapters 11 and 12) that invasion of the body by a parasite generally results in local tissue reactions and the appearance of antibody in the host serum.   It must be emphasised, however, that the appearance of antibody in the serum does not necessarily imply that the resistance of the host has been automatically increased.   This will be the case only if the antibody produced acts on the parasite in such a way as to inhibit its development.   In cestodes, it can do this in a number of ways such as (*a*) by interfering with its relationship to the host tissue, e.g. by stimulating the production of a host capsule (pp. 192-3), (*b*) by producing a precipitate on the microtriches—thus blocking the metabolic process taking place at or in the tegument (e.g. absorption and excretion), or (*c*) by reacting with, and interfering with, glandular secretions from the parasite.

Antibodies which confer a measure of protection on a host are known as 'protective' antibodies and the antigens which stimulate their production are sometimes referred to as 'functional' or 'essential' antigens.   Such antigens are essential to the proper functioning of a parasite, and if the processes in which they are concerned are attacked or modified in some way by antibody, the parasite can no longer survive.

Acquired resistance, based on the production of 'protective' antibodies, can be produced in two ways:

(1) *Actively*:

(*a*) *Naturally,* as a result of a natural infection with either

(i) a parasite of the same species (homologous);
or   (ii) a parasite of a different species (heterologous).

(*b*) *Artificially,* after injection of:

(i) endogenous ('somatic') vaccines, i.e. extracts or homogenates of cestode tissues;

(ii) exogenous (' metabolic ') vaccines, i.e. excretions, secretions or metabolites of cestodes;

(iii) ' live ' vaccines i.e. larval or adult cestodes attenuated (weakened by physical treatments such as irradiation).

(2) *Passively*:

by transfer of antibodies in injected antiserum.

Virtually all the work on both naturally (and artificially) acquired immunity has been carried out on the Cyclophyllidea. Some of these species, especially *Hymenolepis nana*, represent elegant experimental models which particularly lend themselves to studies in this field. A number of reviews are available.[118, 154, 211, 381, 435, 436, 458, 475]

Naturally Acquired Immunity

In the Intermediate Host

General account. Most work in this field has centred on species whose larvae develop in the tissues of mammals. The most studied larvae have been those of *H. nana* and *Hydatigera taeniaeformis* in rodents, *T. pisiformis* in rabbits, *T. saginata* in cattle, *T. hydatigena* in sheep, *Echinococcus* spp., in various hosts. These species make intimate contact with the tissues of the host at two sites, the first, during the early phase of infection when the recently-hatched oncosphere, penetrates the intestine and the second, at the final encystment site where this is a visceral site, such as the liver (e.g. *Echinococcus*) or villi (e.g. *H. nana*). It is not surprising, therefore, to find that a high degree of acquired resistance to reinfection is common for these forms. Indeed, in some cases this approaches a degree of absolute immunity, which furthermore, may persist for long periods.[475] A further remarkable feature is the rapidity (within nine hours) with which this acquired resistance may develop to effective levels. High levels of resistance are not always developed, however, and in some cases, e.g. *Echinococcus*, only moderate levels of resistance may be developed. The acquired immunity patterns of individual species are discussed below.

Hydatigera taeniaeformis (larva: *Cysticercus fasciolaris*). This species was the first to which acquired immunity in the intermediate host was convincingly demonstrated.[244] It was shown that rats with infections of some weeks duration of *Cysticercus fasciolaris* were immune to a challenge infection of oncospheres of the same species. This protection persisted for at least sixty days, even after encapsulated larvae were removed from the rat liver.[246] It is clear that in this case, the oncospheres are eliminated either at the intestinal site or during the process of migration from this site to the final visceral site. The immune mechanisms, which may be due to tissue reactions or antibody reactions or to combinations of both, are said to induce ' early ' or ' pre-encystment ' immunity.[118] An ' early ' antibody has been detected in relation to this phase.[435] This result is in contrast with immune effects which operate after a larva becomes established in its definitive site; this has been termed ' late ', or ' post-encystment ', immunity[118] (see below).

Taenia spp. A similar pattern has been reported for several other larval *Taenia* species—*T. pisiformis*,[196] *T. saginata*,[437] and *T. hydatigena*.[443] In the case of *C. bovis* (*T. saginata*) at least, the immunity is developed both at the ' pre- ' and ' post-encystment ' phases. Although antibodies have been detected during the course of *C. bovis* infections,[435] the nature of this immunity has not been determined. In this species too, both the size of the initial immunising infection and also the age of the host appear to be important factors in determining the levels of immunity developed.

Echinococcus spp. Absolute immunity against the cystic form of *Echinococcus* does not occur, although partial resistance develops; there is also great individual variation, both dead and viable cysts occurring in the same organ.[116] In some sheep, no live cysts occur, in others 100% may be viable although antibodies are present.[444]

The immunological picture in *Echinococcus* may prove to be exceptionally complicated for two reasons. Firstly, the host reaction against this species is characterised by the laying down of a thick laminated membrane round the parasite. If this is laid down sufficiently rapidly, it may prevent further antibodies from reaching the developing cyst, which can thus continue to grow. On the other hand, if antibody reaches the organism before it becomes walled off by the cyst wall, it may affect it sufficiently to kill it. Secondly, the situation is complicated by the fact that the hermaphrodite characteristic of cestodes (pp. 4-5), combined with polyembryony (in *Echinoccocus*), particularly lends itself to the production of numerous ' strains ' (clones) of the same species (Chapter 1). Therefore, it may be that those cysts which become established, are developed from eggs of a ' strain ' which are immunologically adapted to that particular host. In contrast, cysts which fail to survive could represent those from eggs not immunologically adapted to that host.[433]

That some degree of ' post-encystment ' immunity to *E. granulosus* can develop, however, is shown by vaccination experiments described later (p. 222).

Hymenolepis nana. This species has been extensively used as a classical experimental model for studies in cestode immunity. The basic data on acquired resistance to this species were established by early workers;[176, 382] their results, together with the extensive literature of more recent workers, are summarised in recent reviews.[118, 154, 211, 435, 475]

Briefly, the immunological picture of *H. nana* appears to be as follows. When mice are fed eggs and later challenged with a further dose of eggs it has been shown[147, 153] that the immunity (*a*) is probably discernible as early as nine hours after the initial infection, (*b*) reaches an effective level at twelve hours, and (*c*) becomes absolute after twenty-four hours (Table 40); moreover this immunity remains absolute for at least 163 days. In some mice, a few challenge eggs may hatch, penetrate and develop to the cysticercoid stage within the villi, but none develop to adults. This immunity appears to be the result of two processes: (*a*) an initial rapid response in the mucosal cells, which makes oncosphere penetration difficult or impossible and (*b*) a later, more typical, tissue reaction which walls off and kills any larvae that succeed in penetrating.[20]

In this immune process, the reaction of the secretions of the penetration glands in the oncosphere with antibody may be an important factor. Natural passive immunity, i.e. via the mother, has also been demonstrated (p. 221). Antibodies are demonstrable in infected mice serum by means of precipitation, complement fixation, and agglutination tests.[435]

The degree of immunity discussed above develops as a result of an egg immunising dose, followed by an egg challenging dose. If the former is followed, instead, by a cysticercoid challenge dose (i.e. from infected beetles), only about one-fifth as many adults develop as in controls receiving no egg immunisation. Thus, some degree of inhibition to a lumen infection by the preceding tissue infection has been demonstrated.[154] When a cysticercoid immunising dose was followed by an egg challenge, a substantial degree of immunity against development in the host villi, and subsequently against adult worms in the intestine, developed. In contrast, a cysticercoid immunisation followed by a cysticercoid challenge dose, does not result in the development of immunity against establishment in the lumen.

Immunity to *H. nana* is apparently reduced by injections of testosterone and increased by injections of oestradiol.[19] There is also evidence of a degree of cross immunity by *H. diminuta*, *H. microstoma* or *H. citelli* against challenging egg infections of *H. nana*.[474-5]

In the Definitive Host

Adult cestodes, being intestinal parasites, are generally considered to be poorly immunogenic, although the evidence is somewhat conflicting.[118, 435, 475]   Clearly, unless the scolex contact with the intestinal mucosa is very intimate, sufficient antigenic stimulus to the host will not be provided.   As has been shown elsewhere (p. 197) in species such as *Dipylidium caninum* or *E. granulosus* in dogs, or *Aploparaxis furcigera* and *Hymenolepis parvula* in birds, the intestinal mucosa cells are sometimes flattened or even broken down, so that a fairly intimate contact can be established.   The contact is also fairly intimate in the case of *H. nana* (Fig. 6).   In the case of *E. granulosus*, during the early stages of infection, while the protoscoleces are still small, even the lamina propria may be invaded.   Nevertheless, the level of serum antibody detected in adult infections is generally low.[79, 435]

In general, however, lumen-dwelling cestodes do not evoke reactions which protect against reinfection,[475] and no acquired resistance appears to be evoked by *H. taeniaeformis, T. saginata, M. expansa, R. cesticillus.*[118, 435]

In the case of adult *H. diminuta*, an inhibitory effect has been observed on challenge with a new infection, but parasite crowding, and competition for nutrients between worms, may be sufficient to account for this apparent acquired resistance.[475]

Repeated (more than five) infections of *E. granulosus* appear to induce some degree of immunity to this species in some dogs, as evidenced by a reduction in numbers of worms or a decrease in growth, or both.[118]   The effect was not, however, produced in all dogs and did not persist for long periods.

The position with regard to *H. nana* is complicated by the invasion of the villi by hatched oncospheres in direct egg infections.   The general conclusion from a number of studies[20, 151-3, 475] appears to be that no resistance is acquired as the result of a single infection of the lumen-dwelling form (i.e. a cysticercoid from an insect intermediate host), but a partial resistance to this stage develops in mice previously exposed to the tissue-invading larva.   Autoinfection appears to be possible only when the lumen-dwelling form infects the intestine before the tissue forms.

It has already been pointed out that, although some serum antibodies are developed against *H. nana*,[78, 80] they have little apparent effect on the adult worms.   In contrast, mucosal extract[475] gives a typical serological reaction with live worms; which suggests that some antibody leaks into the lumen from the mucosal cells.

Artificially Acquired Immunity (Vaccination)

General Considerations

The realisation, that acquired immunity to diseases of helminth origin can develop, has led to increased efforts to develop vaccines against metazoan parasites. Although some success has been achieved with nematodes, only very modest success has been achieved with trematodes[422] and cestodes.

As shown below, some degree of success can be achieved by passive immunisation using antisera. Most vaccination attempts have used antigenic materials prepared in one of the following ways.

(i) Homogenised fresh or dried adults, eggs or larval stages or fluids or extracts of these or formalin-killed material of the same stages; both homologous and heterologous species have been used,

(ii) Living eggs or larval stages of heterologous species are used.

(iii) metabolic products (i.e. exoantigens) from adults or larvae are used.

(iv) attenuated eggs or larval stages are used.

Passive (Transfer) Immunity

The high degree of immunity developed against *Cysticercus fasciolaris* and *C. pisiformis* can be transmitted to rodents by passive transfer.[196, 245] There is evidence [475] that the protective properties of immune serum in passive transport alters in character with the progress of the donor infection. Serum taken during the second week of infection was protective against the pre-encystment phase but serum taken some weeks later was mainly effective against established larvae, i.e. the post-encystment phase. Passive immunity has also been reported for *H. nana* and may be transmitted from infected mothers to offspring.[147, 209]

Active Immunity

General considerations. Although it is relatively easy to vaccinate against several species of larval cestodes in laboratory animals, vaccination against important human pathogens, such as *Echinococcus* or against adult cestodes has not been very successful.

Vaccination with killed or homogenised tissue. Strobilate tissue, or crude homogenates of it, or cystic tissue, killed eggs, or hydatid cyst fluid, have all been used as antigens in attempts to vaccinate, particularly against larval stages. Homogenates of strobila or cyst material have been shown to provide partial protection against *H. taeniaeformis*.[118] Most of the protection appears to be directed against the post-encystment phase.

Similar results have been obtained with *H. nana* following the repeated use of fresh adult-worm antigen;[210] the degree of immunity produced was not as great as in natural infections, a result probably due to the greater release of metabolic materials in the latter instance. A substantial degree of protection has been induced against *Cysticercus pisiformis* in rabbits by the use of dried worm materials.[196] The degree of immunity varied from partial to complete. As is evidenced from Table 43, immunity again was directed against the ' post-encystment ' phase. Control animals were heavily infected.

TABLE 43

Vaccination of rabbits against Cysticercus pisiformis *using six intraperitoneal injections of dried worms ;* 10 *rabbits in each group*

(Data from Kerr[196])

	Average number of worms				
	Living larvae			Total living	Total dead larvae
	Small	large	migrating		
Vaccinated :					
Autopsy : 21 days	2·6	2·0	0	4·6	7·2
Autopsy : 42 days	0	3·6	3·2	6·8	6·0
Control :	31·4	53·9	94·1	179·4	7·3

A number of attempts have been made to vaccinate both sheep and dogs against the cystic and strobilar phase of *E. granulosus*, using dried protoscoleces and germinal membranes—extracts of these or hydatid fluid.[112, 421] In the cystic stage, no protection appears to be developed against the ' pre-encystment ' stage, but some protection against the ' post-encystment ' stage has been reported. Some success with the vaccination of dogs against *E. granulosus* has been claimed;[105] immunised dogs were said to have smaller worm burdens than controls, and the antibody titre to be in proportion to the antigen used. This is an interesting result and, if confirmed by later work may support the view (p. 220) that some resistance against lumen-dwelling adults can develop. This mechanism may operate via antibodies in the mucus, or sufficient antibodies may leak through tissues from the broken or distended crypt walls (Figs. 12, 73).

The use of larval antigens appears to be an anomaly as it might be expected that antigens from *adult* material might induce better protection. Some success has been obtained by vaccination of dogs with powdered, frozen-dried adults worms and with oncospheres.[112] Although some worms developed in all except one of the dogs vaccinated, there was a general retardation, and in some cases complete arrest, of the maturation of the terminal segments. This result suggests that antibodies against some functional antigen controlling growth were developed, possibly the surface of the microtriches in the tegument may have been blocked with consequent inhibition of nutrient or gaseous transport. Inactivation of the rostellar gland may also be involved. It has been shown (Fig. 85) that precipitations occur on adult *Echinococcus* in serum from infected dogs, a result which strongly points to an antigen-antibody reaction.

Vaccination with living tissue. In contrast to the results with dried material (p. 221) injections of living strobilar material of *H. taeniae-formis* into the abdominal cavity of rats, gave complete immunity to an oral egg challenge at the ' pre-encystment ' level.[118] No protection was developed against a challenge infection of *H. nana* made by using a comparable technique with living strobilar tissue injected intra-peritoneally.[147] The difference between these results may indicate that the immune mechanism to this species is located in the villi; alternatively the short length of the oncosphere migration route in *H. nana* (Fig. 1) may not be sufficient to ' boost ' the immunity to an effective level.

Unhatched eggs and artificially hatched and activated embryos have proved to be promising antigens. This is probably related to the fact that, in the Taeniidae at least, many species appear to share antigens. A series of extended studies have been carried out on *T. ovis*, *T. hydatigena*, *T. pisiformis* and *E. granulosus*.[113-117]

Results of these experiments are summarised in Table 44. In summary, they show that injections of eggs of homologous or heterologous species may confer a marked degree of protection both at the early (i.e. pre-encystment) and later (i.e. post-encystment) levels. In many cases, this immunity is absolute, although its longevity has not been determined; in others no immunity is developed. Thus, activated embryos of *T. hydatigena* gave virtually 100% protection against this species at the pre-encystment and post-encystment level. In contrast, live eggs of *T. pisiformis* gave no protection whatsoever against a challenge of *T. hydatigena*, *T. ovis* or *E. granulosus* (Table 44) although giving substantial protection against the homologous species. Some degree of protection is also given by oncosphere vaccines of heterologous species against the adult stages of *E. granulosus* in dogs; protection was not, however, absolute in all dogs.[118]

Since the living eggs or activated embryos produce a much greater protection than dead eggs,[113] part at least of the antigen complex probably concerned in this protection may be a metabolite produced by the oncosphere, or one released from the oncosphere shortly after injection. Attention has already been drawn (p. 207) to the probable antigenic properties of the so-called ' penetration glands ', and it is possible that by culturing oncospheres *in vitro*, the exoantigens may be collected and concentrated and more effective vaccines thereby developed.

It has been speculated[117] that there are at least two functional groups of antigens in oncospheres. The first is believed to be species-specific

TABLE 44

The percentage efficiency of homologous and heterologous eggs and activated embryos as vaccines in protecting intermediate hosts against the establishment and subsequent survival of the cystic stages of various Taenia *species*

(Data modified from Gemmell[113–116])

Vaccine		Challenge infection with :							
		T. hydatigena		*T. pisiformis*		*T. ovis*		*E. granulosus*	
Parasite	Antigen	Immunity		Immunity		Immunity		Immunity	
		Early*	Late†	Early	Late	Early	Late	Early	Late
T. hydatigena	Emb.	99·9	100	28·0	48·6	48·0	10·7	31·3	89·0
	Eggs	71·3	99·5	19·2	0·0	54·3	51·8	0·0	6·9
T. ovis	Emb.	51·0	100	45·1	25·1	85·5	94·6	38·4	97·4
	Eggs	39·7	8·7	0·0	8·7	55·6	94·7	19·8	0·0
T. pisiformis	Emb.	23·0	35·0	92·4	88·8	0·0	0·0	0·0	19·3
	Eggs	22·5	0·0	97·9	58·5	21·6	0·0	0·0	0·0
E. granulosus	Emb.	—	—	—	—	—	—	91·2	96·0
	Eggs	—	—	—	—	—	—	91·9	100

* at the intestinal level.
† at the site of election.

and contained in the viable egg of the homologous species; this complex induces immunity during the initial invasion of the mucosa. The second antigen complex, present in the activated embryos of several species of different genera, is believed to exert its effect chiefly against the post-encystment phase at the site of election.

It is clear that the successful vaccination of man or domestic animals against diseases of cestode origin (such as hydatidiasis) is likely to come only after a detailed analysis, by advanced immunological methods, of the composition and origin of antigens and metabolites produced by all stages of cestodes—eggs, larvae and adults. Moreover, these studies will need to be supplemented further by cytological studies of the histopathology of the infected hosts.   In addition, the use of *in vitro* cultivation, both for isolation of antigens and for the determination of the precise effect of antibodies on the parasite, is likely to assume increasing importance.

Quite apart from their parasitological value, such studies may have considerable intrinsic interest and raise fundamental questions common to other areas of biology, at a molecular, cellular, tissue and whole organism level.

References

1. AGOSIN, M. 1957. Studies on the metabolism of *Echinococcus granulosus*. II. Some observations on the carbohydrate metabolism of hydatid cyst scolices. *Expl Parasit.*, **6**: 586-593.
2. — 1959. Biquimica de *Echinococcus granulosus*. *Biologica*, **28**: 3-32.
3. AGOSIN, M. and ARAVENA, L. 1959. Studies on the metabolism of *Echinococcus granulosus*. III. Glycolysis, with special reference to hexokinases and related glycolytic enzymes. *Biochim. biophys. Acta*, **34**: 90-102.
4. — 1960a. Studies on the metabolism of *Echinococcus granulosus*. V. The phosphopentose isomerase of hydatid cyst scolices. *Enzymologia*, **22**: 281-294.
5. — 1960b. Studies on the metabolism of *Echinococcus granulosus*. IV. Enzymes of the pentose phosphate pathway. *Expl Parasit.*, **10**: 28-38.
6. AGOSIN, M., VON BRAND, T., RIVERA, G. F. and McMAHON, P. 1957. Studies on the metabolism of *Echinococcus granulosus*. I. General chemical composition and respiratory reactions. *Expl Parasit.*, **6**: 37-51.
7. AGOSIN, M. and REPETTO, Y. 1961. Studies on the metabolism of *Echinococcus granulosus*. VI. Pathways of glucose C^{14} metabolism of *Echinococcus granulosus* scolices. *Biologica*, **32**: 33-38.
8. — 1963. Studies on the metabolism of *Echinococcus granulosus*. VII. Reactions of the tricarboxylic acid cycle in *E. granulosus* scolices. *Comp. Biochem. Physiol.*, **8**: 245-261.
9. — 1965. Studies on the metabolism of *Echinococcus granulosus*. VIII. The pathway to succinate in *E. granulosus* scolices. *Comp. Biochem. Physiol.*, **14**: 299-309.
10. ALDRICH, D. V., CHANDLER, A. C. and DAUGHERTY, J. W. 1954. Intermediary protein metabolism in helminths. II. Effect of host castration on amino acid metabolism in *Hymenolepis diminuta*. *Expl Parasit.*, **3**: 173-184.
11. ALT, H. L. and TISCHER, O. A. 1932. Observations on the metabolism of the tapeworm, *Moniezia expansa*. *Proc. Soc. exp. Biol., N.Y.*, **29**: 222-224.
12. ARCHER, D. M. and HOPKINS, C. A. 1958a. Studies on cestode metabolism. III. Growth pattern of *Diphyllobothrium* sp., in a definitive host. *Expl Parasit.*, **7**: 125-144.
13. — 1958b. Studies on cestode metabolism. V. The chemical composition of *Diphyllobothrium* sp., in the plerocercoid and adult stages. *Expl Parasit.*, **7**: 542-554.
14. ARME, C. 1966. Histochemical and biochemical studies on some enzymes of *Ligula intestinalis* (Cestoda: Pseudophyllidea). *J. Parasit.*, **52**: 63-68.
15. ARME, C. and OWEN, R. W. 1967. Infections of the three-spined stickle-

back *Gasterosteus aculeatus* L., with the plerocercoid larvae of *Schisto-cephalus solidus* (Müller, 1776), with special reference to pathological effects. *Parasitology*, **57**: 301-314.

15a. ARTEMOV, N. M. and LURE, R. N. 1941. [On the content of acetyl-choline and cholinesterase in the tissues of tapeworms.] In Russian, German summary. *Bull. Acad. Sci. URSS* (Sér. Biol.), **2**: 278-282.

16. BAER, J. and JOYEUX, C. 1961. Platyhelminthes, Mésozaires, Acantho-céphales, Nemertiens. In: *Traité de Zoologie*, T. IV. Fasc. 1., 561-692. *Ed.* P. Grassé. Masson et Cie., Paris.

17. BAERNSTEIN, H. D. 1963. A review of electron transport mechanisms in parasitic protozoa. *J. Parasit.*, **49**: 12-21.

18. BAILENGER, J., BAUDOUIN, M. and PAUTRIZEL, R. 1961. Étude de l'immunité des Rongeurs à l'égard d'*Hymenolepis nana*. *Annls. Parasit. hum. comp.*, **36**: 595-610.

19. BAILENGER, J., ROGER, G. and PAUTRIZEL, R. 1964. Étude de l'immunité des Rongeurs à l'égard d'*Hymenolepis nana*. *Annls. Parasit. hum. comp.*, **39**: 33-52.

20. BAILEY, W. S. 1951. Host tissue reactions to initial and super-imposed infection with *Hymenolepis nana* var. *fraterna*. *J. Parasit.*, **37**: 440-444.

21. BAUER, O. N. 1959. [Parasites of freshwater fish and the biological basis for their control.] In Russian. *Bull. State Sci. Res. Inst. Lake River Fisheries, Leningrad*, **49**: 3-215. [English translation Office Tech. Serv., U.S. Dept. Commerce.]

22. BECK, J. W. 1952. Effect of gonadectomy and gonadal hormones on singly established *Hymenolepis diminuta* in rats. *Expl Parasit.*, **1**: 109-117.

23. BÉGUIN, F. 1966. Étude au microscope électronique de la cuticle et de ses structures associées chez quelques cestodes. Essai d'histologie comparée. *Z. Zellforsch. mikrosk. Anat.*, **72**: 30-46.

24. BELL, E. J. and SMYTH, J. D. 1958. Cytological and histochemical criteria for evaluating development of trematodes and pseudophyllidean cestodes *in vivo* and *in vitro*. *Parasitology*, **48**: 131-148.

25. BERNTZEN, A. K. 1961. The *in vitro* cultivation of tapeworms. I. Growth of *Hymenolepis diminuta* (Cestoda: Cyclophyllidea). *J. Parasit.*, **47**: 351-355.

26. — 1962. *In vitro* cultivation of tapeworms. II. Growth and maintenance of *Hymenolepis nana* (Cestoda: Cyclophyllidea). *J. Parasit.*, **48**: 785-797.

27. — 1966. A controlled culture environment for axenic growth of parasites. *Ann. N.Y. Acad. Sci.*, **139**: 176-189.

28. — 1967. Monoxenic cultivation of *Hymenolepis nana* cysticercoids with rat fibroblast cells. Unpublished work.

29. BERNTZEN, A. K. and MUELLER, J. F. 1964. *In vitro* cultivation of *Spirometra mansonoides* (Cestoda) from the procercoid to the early adult. *J. Parasit.*, **50**: 705-711.

30. BERNTZEN, A. K. and VOGE, M. 1962. *In vitro* hatching of oncospheres of *Hymenolepis nana* and *Hymenolepis citelli* (Cestoda: Cyclophyllidea). *J. Parasit.*, **48**: 110-119.

228 THE PHYSIOLOGY OF CESTODES

30a. BERNTZEN, A. K. and VOGE, M. 1965. *In vitro* hatching of oncospheres of four hymenolepidid cestodes. *J. Parasit.*, **51**: 235-242.
31. BIGUET, J., CAPRON, A. and KY, P. TRAN VAN. 1962. Les antigènes de *Fasciola hepatica*. Étude électrophorétique identification des fractions et comparaison avec antigènes correspondant à sept autres Helminthes. *Annls. Parasit. hum. comp.*, **37**: 221-231.
32. BOGITSH, B. J. 1963. Histochemical studies on *Hymenolepis microstoma* (Cestoda: Hymenolepididae). *J. Parasit.*, **49**: 989-997.
33. BOGOMOPOVA, N. A. and CHAVPOVA, P. E. 1961. [Vitelline cells of *Fasciola hepatica* and *Diphyllobothrium latum* and their role in the formation of the egg shell and nutrition of the embryo.] *Helminthologia*, **3**: 47-59. (In Russian, English summary)
34. BRAND, T. VON. 1952. *Chemical physiology of endoparasitic animals.* Academic Press, N.Y.
35. — 1960. Recent advances in carbohydrate biochemistry of helminths. *Helminth. Abstr.*, **29**: 1-15.
36. — 1966. *Biochemistry of Parasites.* Academic Press, N.Y.
37. BRAND, T. VON and ALLING, D. W. 1962. Relations between size and metabolism in larval and adult *Taenia taeniaeformis*. *Comp. Biochem. Physiol.*, **5**: 141-148.
38. BRAND, T. VON and BOWMAN, I. B. R. 1961. Studies on the aerobic and anaerobic metabolism of larval and adult *Taenia taeniaeformis*. *Expl Parasit.*, **11**: 276-297.
39. BRAND, T. VON, CHURCHILL, F. and HIGGINS, H. 1966. Aerobic and anaerobic metabolism of larval and adult *Taenia taeniaeformis*. IV. Absorption of glycerol; relations between glycerol absorption and glucose absorption and leakage. *Expl Parasit.*, **19**: 110-123.
40. BRAND, T. VON and GIBBS, E. 1966. Aerobic and anaerobic metabolism of larval and adult *Taenia taeniaeformis*. III. Influence of some cations on glucose uptake, glucose leakage and tissue glucose. *Proc. helminth. Soc. Wash.*, **33**: 1-4.
41. BRAND, T. VON, MCMAHON, P., GIBBS, E. and HIGGINS, H. 1964. Aerobic and anaerobic metabolism of larval and adult *Taenia taeniaeformis*. II. Hexose leakage and absorption; tissue glucose and polysaccharides. *Expl Parasit.*, **15**: 410-429.
42. BRAND, T. VON, MERCADO, T. I., NYLEN, M. U. and SCOTT, D. B. 1960. Observations on function, composition and structure of cestode calcareous corpuscles. *Expl Parasit.*, **9**: 205-214.
43. BRAND, T. VON, NYLEN, M. U., SCOTT, D. B. and MARTIN, G. N. 1965. Observations on calcareous corpuscles of larval *Echinococcus granulosus* of various geographic origins. *Proc. Soc. exp. Biol. Med.*, **120**: 383-385.
44. BRAND, T. VON, SCOTT, D. B., NYLEN, M. R. and PUGH, M. H. 1965. Variations in the mineralogical composition of cestode calcareous corpuscles. *Expl Parasit.*, **16**: 382-391.
45. BRAND, T. VON and WEINBACH, E. C. 1965. Incorporation of phosphate into the soft tissues and calcareous corpuscles of larval *Taenia taeniaeformis*. *Comp. Biochem. Physiol.*, **14**: 11-20.

46. BRUNET, P. C. J. 1967. Sclerotins. *Endeavour* **26**: 68-74.

47. BRYANT, C. and MORSETH, D. J. 1968. The metabolism of radioactive fumaric acid and some other substrates by whole adult *Echinococcus granulosus* (Cestoda). *Comp. Biochem. Physiol.* **25**: 541-546.

48. BUEDING, E. 1962. Comparative aspects of carbohydrate metabolism. *Proc. Fedn Am. Socs exp. Biol.*, **21**: 1039-1046.

49. BURTON, P. R. 1964. The ultrastructure of the integument of the frog lung-fluke, *Haematoloechus medioplexus* (Trematoda: Plagiorchiidae). *J. Morph.*, **115**: 305-318.

50. CAMPBELL, D. H., GARVEY, J. S., CREMER, N. E. and SUSSDORF, D. H. 1963. *Methods in Immunology*. W. A. Benjamin, Inc., N.Y.

51. CAMPBELL, J. W. 1960a. Pyrimidine metabolism in parasitic flatworms. *Biochem. J.*, **77**: 105-112.

52. — 1960b. Nitrogen and amino acid composition of three species of anoplocephalid cestodes: *Moniezia expansa, Thysanosoma actinioides* and *Cittotaenia perplexa*. *Expl Parasit.*, **9**: 1-8.

53. — 1963a. Urea formation and urea cycle enzymes in the cestode, *Hymenolepis diminuta*. *Comp. Biochem. Physiol.*, **8**: 13-27.

54. — 1963b. Amino acids and nucleotides of the cestode, *Hymenolepis diminuta*. *Comp. Biochem. Physiol.*, **8**: 181-185.

55. CAMPBELL, J. W. and LEE, T. W. 1963. Ornithine transcarbamylase and arginase activity in flatworms. *Comp. Biochem. Physiol.*, **8**: 29-38.

56. CAMPBELL, W. C. 1963. The efficiency of surface-active agents in stimulating the evagination of cysticerci *in vitro*. *J. Parasit.*, **49**: 81-84.

57. CHANDLER, A. C., READ, C. P. and NICHOLAS, H. O. 1950. Observations on certain phases of nutrition and host-parasite relations of *Hymenolepis diminuta* in white rats. *J. Parasit.*, **36**: 523-535.

58. CHEAH, K. S. 1967a. Spectrophotometric studies on the succinate oxidase system of *Taenia hydatigena*. *Comp. Biochem. Physiol.*, **20**: 867-875.

59. — 1967b. Histochemical and spectrophotometric demonstration of peroxidase in *Moniezia expansa* (Cestoda). *Comp. Biochem. Physiol.*, **21**: 351-355.

60. — 1967c. Studies on the oxidative metabolism of *Moniezia expansa* (Cestoda). Ph.D. Thesis. Australian National University, Canberra.

61. — 1967d. The oxidase systems of *Moniezia expansa*. *Comp. Biochem. Physiol.*, **23**: 277-302.

62. CHEAH, K. S. and BRYANT, C. 1966. Studies on the electron transport system of *Moniezia expansa* (Cestoda). *Comp. Biochem. Physiol.*, **19**: 197-223.

63. CHEN, H. T. 1934. Reactions of *Ctenocephalides felis* to *Dipylidium caninum*. *Z. ParasitKde*, **6**: 603-637.

64. — 1950. The *in vitro* action of rat immune serum on the larvae of *Taenia taeniaeformis*. *J. infect. Dis.*, **86**: 205-213.

65. CHENG, T. C. and DYCKMAN, E. 1964. Sites of glycogen deposition in *Hymenolepis diminuta* during the growth phase in rodents. *Z ParasitKde*, **24**: 27-48.

66. CHORDI, A. and KAGAN, I. G. 1965. Identification and characterization

of antigenic components of sheep hydatid fluid by immunoelectrophoresis. *J. Parasit.*, **51**: 63-71.

67. CHOWDHURY, A. B. 1955. Histological and histochemical observations on *Taenia saginata*. *Bull. Calcutta Sch. trop. Med. Hyg.*, **3**: 143-144.

68. CHOWDHURY, A. B., DASGUPTA, B. and RAY, H. N. 1962. On the nature and structure of the calcareous corpuscles in *Taenia saginata*. *Parasitology*, **52**: 153-157.

69. CLARKE, A. S. 1954. Studies on the life cycle of the pseudophyllidean cestode *Schistocephalus solidus*. *Proc. zool. Soc. Lond.*, **124**: 257-302.

70. CLEGG, J. A. 1965. Secretion of lipoprotein by Mehlis' gland in *Fasciola hepatica*. *Ann. N.Y. Acad. Sci.*, **118**: 969-986.

71. CLEGG, J. A. and MORGAN, J. 1966. The lipid composition of the lipoprotein membranes on the egg-shell of *Fasciola hepatica*. *Comp. Biochem. Physiol.*, **18**: 573-588.

72. CLEGG, J. A. and SMYTH, J. D. 1968. Growth, development, and culture methods: parasitic platyhelminths. In: *Chemical Zoology*, Vol. II. Chapter 5, pp. 395-446. Academic Press, London & New York.

73. ČMELIK, S. 1952a. Ein antigenes Polysaccharid aus den Echinococcuscyten. *Biochem. Z.*, **322**: 456-462.

74. — 1952b. Zur Kenntnis der Lipoide aus den Cystenmembranen von *Taenia echinococcus*. *Hoppe-Seyler's Z. physiol. Chem.*, **289**: 78-79.

75. — 1955. Novi tip nukleoproteida iz *Taenia echinococcus*. *Glasnik. Hrv. Prirodoslov. Drůstva, Zagreb*, **7**: 123-124.

76. ČMELIK, S. and BARTL, Z. 1956. Zusammensetzung der Lipide von *Taenia saginata*. *Hoppe-Seyler's Z. physiol. Chem.*, **305**: 170-176.

77. ČMELIK, S. and BRISKI, B. 1953. Untersuchungen über Eiweissfraktionen von *Taenia echinococcus*. *Biochem. Z.*, **324**: 104-114.

78. COLEMAN, R. M. 1961. *In vivo* binding sites in *Hymenolepis nana* as demonstrated by direct and indirect immunofluorescent staining. *J. Parasit.*, **47**: (suppl.): 54.

79. COLEMAN, R. M. and DE SA, L. M. 1964. Host response to implanted adult *Hymenolepis nana*. *J. Parasit.*, **50** (suppl.): 17.

80. COLEMAN, R. M. and FOTORNY, N. M. 1962. *In vivo* isolation of *Hymenolepis nana* and antibody-binding sites. *Nature, Lond.*, **195**: 920-921.

81. COLEMAN, R. M., VENUTA, F. X. and FIMIAN, W. J. JN. 1967. Secretion and immunogenicity of dwarf tapeworm esterases. *Nature, Lond.*, **214**: 593-594.

82. COLLINGS, S. B. and HUTCHINS, C. P. 1965. Motility and hatching of *Hymenolepis microstoma* oncospheres in sera, beetle extracts and salines. *Expl Parasit.*, **16**: 53-56.

83. CROMPTON, D. W. T. 1966. Measurements of glucose and amino acid concentrations, temperature and pH in the habitat of *Polymorphus minutus* (Acanthocephala) in the intestine of domestic ducks. *J. exp. Biol.*, **45**: 279-284.

84. CROMPTON, D. W. T., SHRIMPTON, D. H. and SILVER, I. A. 1965. Measurements of the oxygen tension in the lumen of the small intestine of the domestic duck. *J. exp. Biol.*, **43**: 473-478.

85. CROWLE, A. J. 1961. *Immunodiffusion*. Academic Press, N.Y.
86. DAUGHERTY, J. W. 1954. Synthesis of amino nitrogen from ammonia in *Hymenolepis diminuta*. *Proc. Soc. exper. Biol. Med.*, **85**: 288-291.
87. — 1955. Intermediary protein metabolism in helminths. III. The l-amino acid oxidases in *Hymenolepis diminuta* and some effects of changes in host physiology. *Expl Parasit.*, **4**: 455-463.
88. — 1957a. Intermediary protein metabolism in helminths. IV. The active absorption of methionine by the cestode, *H. diminuta*. *Expl Parasit.*, **6**: 60-67.
89. — 1957b. The active absorption of certain metabolites by helminths. *Amer. J. trop. Med. Hyg.*, **6**: 464-470.
90. DAUGHERTY, J. W. and FOSTER, W. B. 1958. Comparative studies on amino acid absorption by cestodes. *Expl Parasit.*, **7**: 99-107.
91. DAVENPORT, H. W. 1966. *Physiology of the digestive tract*. Year Bk. Medical Pub. Inc., Chicago.
91a. DAVEY, K. G. and BRECKENRIDGE, W. R. 1967. Neurosecretory cells in a cestode, *Hymenolepis diminuta*. *Science*, **158**: 931-932.
92. DAVIES, P. S. and WALKEY, M. 1966. The effect of body size and temperature upon oxygen consumption of the cestode *Schistocephalus solidus* (Müller). *Comp. Biochem. Physiol.*, **18**: 415-425.
93. DIXON, M. and WEBB, E. C. 1964. *Enzymes*. 2nd Ed., Longmans, Green, London.
94. DOUGLAS, L. T. 1963. The development of organ systems in nemato-taeniid cestodes. III. Gametogenesis and embryonic development in *Baerietta diana* and *Distoichometra kozloffi*. *J. Parasit.*, **49**: 530-558.
95. DUBININA, M. N. 1960. On the possibility of progenesis in plerocercoids of the family Ligulidae (Cestoda). *Zool. Zh.*, **39**: 1467-1477.
96. DUNNING, W. F. and CURTIS, M. R. 1953. Attempts to isolate the active agent in *Cysticercus fasciolaris*. *Cancer Res.*, **13**: 838-842.
97. DVORAK, J. A. and JONES, A. W. 1963. *In vivo* incorporation of tritiated cytosine and tritiated thymidine by the cestode, *Hymenolepis microstoma*. *Expl Parasit.*, **14**: 316-322.
98. ENIGK, K. and STICINSKY, E. 1957. Über die Bohrdrüsen der Onko-sphäre von *Davainea proglottina* (Cestoidea). *Z. ParasitKde.*, **18**: 48-54.
99. ERASMUS, D. A. 1957a. Studies on phosphatase systems of cestodes. I. Studies on *Taenia pisiformis* (cysticercus and adult). *Parasitology*, **47**: 70-80.
100. — 1957b. Studies on phosphatase systems of cestodes. II. Studies on *Cysticercus tenuicollis* and *Moniezia expansa* (adult). *Parasitology*. **47**: 81-91.
101. FAIRBAIRN, D., WERTHEIM, G., HARPUR, R. P. and SCHILLER, E. L. 1961. Biochemistry of normal and irradiated strains of *Hymenolepis diminuta*. *Expl Parasit.*, **11**: 248-263.
102. FARHAN, I., SCHWABE, C. W. and ZOBEL, C. R. 1959. Host-parasite relationships in echinococcosis. III. Relation of environmental oxygen tension to the metabolism of hydatid scolices. *Am. J. trop. Med. Hyg.*, **8**: 473-477.

103. FAROOQI, H. U. 1958. The occurrence of certain specialised glands in the rostellum of *Taenia solium* L. *Z. ParasitKde.*, **18**: 308-311.
104. FERNEX, M. and FERNEX, P. 1962. Increased number of mast cells and helminthic diseases. Experimental mastocytosis in mice. *Acta trop.*, **19**: 248-251.
105. FORŠEK, Z. and RUKAVINA, J. 1959. [Experimental immunization of dogs against *Echinococcus granulosus*. I. First observations.] *Veterinaria, Saraj.*, **8**: 479-482.
106. FOSTER, W. B. and DAUGHERTY, J. W. 1959. Establishment and distribution of *Raillietina cesticillus* in the fowl and comparative studies on amino acid metabolism of *R. cesticillus* and *Hymenolepis diminuta*. *Expl Parasit.*, **8**: 413-426.
107. FREEMAN, R. S. 1962. Studies on the biology of *Taenia crassiceps* (Zeder, 1800) Rudolphi, 1810 (Cestoda). *Can. J. Zool.*, **40**: 969-990.
108. FRIEDHEIM, E. A. H. and BAER, J. G. 1933. Untersuchungen über die Atmung von *Diphyllobothrium latum* (L). Ein Beitrag zur Kenntnis der Atmungsfermente. *Biochem. Z.*, **265**: 329-337.
109. FROYD, G. and ROUND, M. C. 1960. The artificial infection of adult cattle with *Cysticercus bovis*. *Res. vet. Sci.*, **1**: 275-282.
110. GALLAGHER, I. H. C. 1964. Chemical composition of hooks isolated from hydatid scolices. *Expl Parasit.*, **15**: 110-117.
111. GALLATI, W. W. 1959. Life history, morphology and taxonomy of *Ariotaenia* (*Ershovia*) *procyonis* (Cestoda: Linstowiidae), a parasite of the raccoon. *J. Parasit.*, **45**: 363-377.
112. GEMMELL, M. A. 1962. Natural and acquired immunity factors interfering with development during the rapid growth phase of *Echinococcus granulosus* in dogs. *Immunology*, **5**: 496-503.
113. GEMMELL, M. A. 1964. Immunological responses of the mammalian host against tapeworm infections. I. Species specificity of hexacanth embryos in protecting sheep against *Taenia hydatigena*. *Immunology*, **7**: 489-499.
114. — 1965a. Immunological responses of the mammalian host against tapeworm infections. II. Species specificity of hexacanth embryos in protecting rabbits against *Taenia pisiformis*. *Immunology*, **8**: 270-280.
115. — 1965b. Immunological responses of the mammalian host against tapeworm infections. III. Species specificity of hexacanth embryos in protecting sheep against *Taenia ovis*. *Immunology*, **8**: 281-290.
116. — 1966a. Immunological responses of the mammalian host against tapeworm infections. IV. Species specificity of hexacanth embryos in protecting sheep against *Echinoccus granulosus*. *Immunology*, **11**: 325-335.
117. — 1967. Species specificity and cross-protective functional antigens of the tapeworm embryo. *Nature, Lond.*, **213**: 500-501.
118. GEMMELL, M. A. and SOULSBY, E. J. L. 1968. The development of acquired immunity to tapeworms and progress in research towards active immunization with special reference to *Echinococcus* spp. *Bull. Wld Hlth Org.*, **39**: 45-55.

118a. GERGELY, J. 1964. *Biochemistry of muscle contraction.* Little, Brown & Co., Boston.

119. GINGER, C. D. and FAIRBAIRN, D. 1966a. Lipid metabolism in helminth parasites. I. The lipids of *Hymenolepis diminuta* (Cestoda). *J. Parasit.*, 52: 1086-1096.

120. — 1966b. Lipid metabolism in helminth parasites. II. The major origins of the lipids of *Hymenolepis diminuta* (Cestoda). *J. Parasit.*, 52: 1097-1107.

121. GOLDBERG, E. and NOLF, L. O. 1954. Succinic dehydrogenase activity in the cestode *Hymenolepis nana*. *Expl Parasit.*, 3: 275-284.

122. GÖNNERT, R., MEISTER, G., STRUFE, R. and WEBBE, G. 1967. Biologische Probleme bei *Taenia solium*. *Z. Tropenmed. Parasit.*, 18: 76-81.

123. GOODCHILD, C. G. 1958. Growth and maturation of the cestode *Hymenolepis diminuta* in bileless hosts. *J. Parasit.* 44: 352-362.

124. — 1960. Effects of starvation and lack of bile upon growth, egg production and egg viability in established rat tapeworms, *Hymenolepis diminuta*. *J. Parasit.*, 46: 615-623.

125. — 1961a. Carbohydrate contents of the tapeworm *Hymenolepis diminuta* from normal, bileless and starved rats. *J. Parasit.*, 47: 401-405.

126. — 1961b. Protein contents of the tapeworm *Hymenolepis diminuta* from normal, bileless and starved rats. *J. Parasit.*, 47: 830-832.

127. GOODCHILD, C. G. and DENNIS, E. S. 1966. Amino acids in seven species of cestodes. *J. Parasit.*, 52: 60-62.

128. GOODCHILD, C. G. and HARRISON, D. L. 1961. The growth of the rat tapeworm *Hymenolepis diminuta* during the first five days in the final host. *J. Parasit.*, 47: 819-829.

129. GOODCHILD, C. G. and WELLS, O. C. 1957. Amino acids in larval and adult tapeworms (*Hymenolepis diminuta*) and in the tissues of their rat and beetle hosts. *Expl Parasit.*, 6: 575-585.

130. GRABIEC, S., GUTTOWA, A. and MICHAJŁOW, W. 1963a. Effect of light stimulus on hatching of coracidia of *Diphyllobothrium latum* (L.). *Acta parasit. pol.*, 11: 229-238.

131. — 1963b. Structure of the ciliated envelope of the coracidium of *Diphyllobothrium latum* (L.) (Cestoda, Pseudophyllidea). *Bull. Acad. pol. Sci.*, Cl. II, Sér. Sci. biol., 11: 293-294.

132. — 1964. Investigation on the respiratory metabolism of eggs and coracidia of *Diphyllobothrium latum* (L.) Cestoda. *Bull. Acad. pol. Sci. Cl. II. Sér. Sci. biol.*, 12: 29-34.

133. GRAFF, D. J. and READ, C. P. 1967. Specific acetylcholinesterase in *Hymenolepis diminuta*. *J. Parasit.*, 53: 1030-1031.

134. GREMBERGEN, G. VAN. 1944. Le métabolisme respiratoire du cestode *Moniezia benedeni* (Moniez, 1879). *Enzymologia*, 11: 268-281.

135. GRESSON, R. A. R. 1962. Spermatogenesis of a cestode. *Nature, Lond.*, 194: 397-398.

135a. GURRI, J. 1963. Vitalidad y evolutividad de los escolices hidáticos, *in vivo* e *in vitro*. *An. Fac. Med. Univ. Montevideo*, 48: 372-381.

136. GUTTOWA, A. 1958. Further research on the effect of temperature on

the development of the cestode, *Triaenophotus lucii* (Müll) embryos in eggs, and on the invadability of their oncospheres. *Acta parasit. pol.*, **6**: 367-381.

137. — 1961a. Experimental investigations on the systems ' procercoids of *Diphyllobothrium latum* (L.)—Copepoda '. *Acta parasit. pol.*, **9**: 371-408.

138. — 1961b. Experimental study on ' host-parasite ' relations in ' procercoids *Diphyllobothrium latum* (L.)—Copepoda' systems. *Wiad. parazyt.*, **7**: 217-221.

139. — 1967. Influence of *Triaenophorus nodulosus* (Pall.) (Cestoda) larva on the quantitative occurrence of amino acids in haemolymph of *Eudiaptomus gracilis* (Sars) (Copepoda). *Polish Parasit. Soc. 9th Meeting, Abstracts*: 35-36.

140. HADANO, N. 1959. Studies on the tapeworm antigens. I. *Acta Sch. med. Gifu*, **7**: 808-821.

141. HARLOW, D. R., MERTZ, W. and MUELLER, J. F. 1964. Effects of *Spirometra mansonoides* infection on carbohydrate metabolism. II. An insulin-like activity from the sparganum. *J. Parasit.*, **50**: (Sec. 2) 55.

142. — 1967. Insulin-like activity from the sparganum of *Spirometra mansonoides*. *J. Parasit.*, **53**: 449-454.

143. HARRINGTON, G. W. 1965. The lipid content of *Hymenolepis diminuta* and *Hymenolepis citelli*. *Expl Parasit.*, **17**: 287-295.

144. HART, J. L. 1967. Studies on the nervous system of Tetrathyridia (Cestoda: Mesocestoides). *J. Parasit.*, **53**: 1032-1039.

145. HASKINS, W. T. and OLIVIER, L. 1958. Nitrogenous excretory products of *Taenia taeniaeformis* larvae. *J. Parasit.*, **44**: 569-573.

146. HASLEWOOD, G. A. D. 1967. *Bile Salts*. Methuen.

147. HEARIN, J. T. 1941. Studies on the acquired immunity to the dwarf tapeworm *Hymenolepis nana var. fraterna*, in the mouse host. *Am. J. Hyg.*, **33**: 71-87.

148. HEATH, D. 1967. Personal communication.

148a. — and SMYTH, J. D. 1968. Unpublished work.

149. HEDRICK, R. M. and DAUGHERTY, J. W. 1957. Comparative histochemical studies on cestodes. I. The distribution of glycogen in *Hymenolepis diminuta* and *Raillietina cesticillus*. *J. Parasit.*, **43**: 497-504.

150. HERCUS, C. E., WILLIAMS, R. J., GEMMELL, M. A. and PARNELL, I. W. 1962. A warning that formalin is not a hydatid ovicide. *Vet. Rec.*, **74**: 1515.

151. HEYNEMAN, D. 1961. Studies on helminth immunity. III. Experimental verification of autoinfection from cysticercoids of *Hymenolepis nana* in the white mouse. *J. infect. Dis.*, **109**: 10-18.

152. — 1962a. Studies on helminth immunity. I. Comparison between lumenal and tissue phases of infection in the white mouse by *Hymenolepis nana* (Cestoda: Hymenolepididae). *Am. J. trop. Med. Hyg.*, **2**: 46-63.

153. — 1962b. Studies on helminth immunity. IV. Rapid onset of resistance by the white mouse against a challenging infection with eggs of *Hymenolepis nana* (Cestoda: Hymenolepididae). *J. Immun.*, **88**: 217-220.

154. — 1963. Host-parasite resistance patterns—some implications from experimental studies with helminths. *Ann. N.Y. Acad. Sci.*, **113**: 114-129.

155. HEYNEMAN, D. and VOGE, M. 1960. Succinic dehydrogenase activity in cysticercoids of *Hymenolepis* (Cestoda: Hymenolepididae) measured by the tetrazolium technique. *Expl Parasit.*, **9**: 14-17.

156. HEYNEMAN, D. and WELSH, J. 1959. Action of homologous antiserum *in vitro* against life cycle stages of *Hymenolepis nana*, the dwarf mouse tapeworm. *Expl Parasit.*, **8**: 119-128.

157. HICKMAN, J. L. 1963. The biology of *Oochoristica vacuolata* Hickman (Cestoda). *Pap. Proc. R. Soc. Tasm.*, **97**: 81-104.

158. HILLIARD, D. K. 1960. Studies on the helminth fauna of Alaska. XXXVIII. The taxonomic significance of eggs and coracidia of some diphyllobothriid cestodes. *J. Parasit.*, **46**: 703-716.

159. HOLMES, J. C. 1961. Effects of concurrent infections on *Hymenolepis diminuta* (Cestoda) and *Moniliformis dubius* (Acanthocephala). I. General effects and comparison with crowding. *J. Parasit.*, **47**: 209-216.

160. — 1962a. Effects of concurrent infections on *Hymenolepis diminuta* (Cestoda) and *Moniliformis dubius* (Acanthocephala). II. Effects on growth. *J. Parasit.*, **48**: 87-96.

161. — 1962b. Effects of concurrent infections on *Hymenolepis diminuta* (Cestoda) and *Moniliformis dubius* (Acanthocephala). III. Effects in hamsters. *J. Parasit.*, **48**: 97-100.

162. HOPKINS, C. A. 1950. Studies on cestode metabolism. I. Glycogen metabolism in *Schistocephalus solidus in vivo*. *J. Parasit.*, **36**: 384-390.

163. — 1951. Studies on cestode metabolism. II. The utilization of glycogen by *Schistocephalus solidus in vitro*. *Expl Parasit.*, **1**: 196-213.

164. — 1959. Seasonal variations in the incidence and development of the cestode *Proteocephalus filicollis* (Rud. 1810) in *Gasterosteus aculeatus* (L. 1766). *Parasitology*, **49**: 529-542.

165. — 1960. Studies on cestode metabolism. VI. Analytical procedures and their application to *Hydatigera taeniaeformis*. *Expl Parasit.*, **9**: 159-166.

166. — 1967. The *in vitro* cultivation of cestodes with particular reference to *Hymenolepis nana*. In: *Problems of in vitro culture*. Ed. A. Taylor. 27-47. Blackwell Sci. Publ., Oxford.

167. HOPKINS, C. A. and CALLOW, L. L. 1965. Methionine flux between a tapeworm (*Hymenolepis diminuta*) and its environment. *Parasitology*, **55**: 653-666.

168. HOPKINS, C. A. and HUTCHISON, W. M. 1958. Studies on cestode metabolism. IV. The nitrogen fraction in the large cat tapeworm, *Hydatigera (Taenia) taeniaeformis*. *Expl Parasit.*, **7**: 349-365.

169. — 1960. Studies on *Hydatigera taeniaeformis*. III. The water content of larval and adult worms. *Expl Parasit.*, **9**: 257-263.

170. HOPKINS, C. A. and McCAIG, M. L. O. 1963. Studies on *Schistocephalus solidus*. I. The correlation of development in the plerocercoid with infectivity to the definitive host. *Expl Parasit.*, **13**: 235-243.

171. HOPKINS, C. A. and SMYTH, J. D. 1951. Notes on the morphology and life history of *Schistocephalus solidus* (Cestoda: Diphyllobothriidae). *Parasitology*, 41: 283-291.

172. HOWELLS, R. E. 1965. Electron-microscope and histochemical studies on the cuticle and subcuticular tissues of *Moniezia expansa*. *Parasitology*, 55: 20P-21P.

173. HUFF, C. G. 1940. Immunity in invertebrates. *Physiol. Rev.*, 20: 68-88.

174. HUFFMAN, J. L. and JONES, A. W. 1962. Hatchability, viability and infectivity of *Hydatigera taeniaeformis* eggs. *Expl Parasit.*, 12: 120-124.

175. HUMPHREY, J. H. and WHITE, R. G. 1964. *Immunology for Students of Medicine*. 2nd Ed. Blackwell, Oxford.

176. HUNNINEN, A. V. 1935. Studies on the life history and host-parasite relations of *Hymenolepis fraterna* (*H. nana* var. *fraterna* Stiles) in white mice. *Amer. J. Hyg.*, 22: 414-443.

177. HUTCHISON, W. M. 1958. Studies on *Hydatigera taeniaeformis*. I. Growth of the larval stage. *J. Parasit.*, 44: 574-582.

178. — 1959. Studies on *Hydatigera (Taenia) taeniaeformis*. II. Growth of the adult phase. *Expl Parasit.*, 8: 557-567.

179. HYMAN, L. H. 1951. *The Invertebrates*. Vol. II. McGraw-Hill Book Co. Inc., N.Y.

180. JACOBSEN, N. S. and FAIRBAIRN, D. 1967. Lipid metabolism in helminth parasites. III. Biosynthesis and interconversion of fatty acids by *Hymenolepis diminuta* (Cestoda). *J. Parasit.*, 53: 355-361.

180a. JANSSENS, P. A. and BRYANT, C. 1969. The ornithine-urea cycle in some parasitic helminths. *Comp. Biochem. Phys.*, (In press.)

181. JARECKA, L. 1961. Morphological adaptations of tapeworm eggs and their importance in the life cycles. *Acta parasit. pol.*, 9: 409-426.

182. — 1964. Cycle évolutif à un seul hôte intérmediaire chez *Bothriocephalus claviceps* (Goeze, 1782) cestode de *Anguilla anguilla* L. *Annls Parasit. hum. comp.*, 39: 149-156.

183. JHA, R. K. and SMYTH, J. D. 1969. Ultrastructure of microtriches in *Echinococcus granulosus*. *Expl Parasit.* (In press.)

184. JOHRI, L. N. 1957. A morphological and histochemical study of egg formation in a cyclophyllidean cestode. *Parasitology*, 47: 21-29.

185. JOHRI, L. N. and SMYTH, J. D. 1956. A histochemical approach to the study of helminth morphology. *Parasitology*, 46: 107-116.

186. KAGAN, I. G. 1963. Seminar on immunity to parasitic helminths. VI Hydatid disease. *Expl Parasit.*, 13: 57-71.

187. KAIPAINEN, W. J. and IKKALA, E. 1959. The metabolic activity of *Diphyllobothrium latum* and its relation to viable ova. *Annls Med. intern. Fenn.*, 48: 191-196.

188. KARNOVSKY, M. J. and ROOTS, L. 1964. A 'direct-coloring' thiocholine method for cholinesterases. *J. Histochem. Cytochem.*, 12: 219-221.

189. KENNEDY, C. R. 1965. The life-history of *Archigetes limnodrili* (Yamaguti) (Cestoda: Caryophyllaeidae) and its development in the invertebrate host. *Parasitology*, 55: 427-437.

190. KENT, N. H. 1947. Étude biochimique sur les protéines des *Moniezia* parasites intestinaux du mouton. *Bull. Soc. neuchâtel. Sci. nat.*, **70**: 85-108.

191. — 1957a. Biochemical studies on the proteins of *Hymenolepis diminuta*. *Expl Parasit.*, **6**: 351-357.

192. — 1957b. Studies on protein complexes in the cestode *Raillietina cesticillus*. *Expl Parasit.*, **6**: 486-490.

193. — 1957c. Aspect biochimique de la spécificité chez les cestodes. In *1st Symposium on host specificity among parasites of vertebrates*, pp. 293-307. Paul Attinger, Neuchâtel.

194. — 1963a. (Organizer). Seminar on immunity to parasitic helminths. (Report of discussion held at School of Hygiene and Public Health, Johns Hopkins University.) *Expl Parasit.*, **13**: 1-82.

195. — 1963b. Immunodiagnosis of helminthic infections. VI. Current and potential value of immunodiagnostic tests employing soluble antigens. *Am. J. Hyg. (Monog. Ser.)*, **22**: 68-90.

196. KERR, K. B. 1935. Immunity against a cestode parasite, *Cysticercus pisiformis*. *Amer. J. Hyg.*, **22**: 169-182.

197. KERR, T. 1948. The pituitary in normal and parasitised roach (*Leuciscus rutilus* Flem). *Q. Jl microsc. Sci.*, **89**: 129-137.

198. KILEJIAN, A. 1966. Permeation of l-proline in the cestode, *Hymenolepis diminuta*. *J. Parasit.*, **52**: 1108-1115.

199. KILEJIAN, A., SAUER, K. and SCHWABE, C. W. 1962. Host-parasite relationships in Echinococcosis. VIII. Infrared spectra and chemical composition of the hydatid cyst. *Expl Parasit.*, **12**: 377-392.

200. KILEJIAN, A., SCHINAZI, L. A. and SCHWABE, C. W. 1961. Host-parasite relationships in Echinococcosis. V. Histochemical observations on *Echinococcus granulosus*. *J. Parasit.*, **47**: 181-188.

201. KIRSCHENBLAT, Y. D. 1951. [Effect of plerocercoids of *Ligula intestinalis* on the hypophysis of the roach.] In Russian. *Priroda, Mosk.*, **3**: 67-68.

202. KISIELEWSKA, K. 1957. Influence of some factors on the survival and invasity of eggs of the tapeworm *Drepanidotaenia lanceolata* (Bloch) and on the further development of larvae from such eggs. *Acta parasit. pol.*, **5**: 585-598.

203. — 1959. Types of Copepoda and *Drepanidotaenia lanceolata* (Bloch) host-parasite systems established experimentally. *Acta parasit. pol.*, **7**: 371-392.

204. KMETEC, E. and BUEDING, E. 1961. Succinic and reduced diphospho-pyridine nucleotide oxidase systems of *Ascaris* muscle. *J. biol. Chem.*, **236**: 584-591.

205. KORC, I., HIERRO, J., LASALVIA, E., FALCO, M. and CALCAGNO, M. 1967. Chemical characterisation of the polysaccharide of the hydatid membrane of *Echinococcus granulosus*. *Expl Parasit.*, **20**: 219-224.

206. KRAUT, N. 1956. An electrophoretic study of sera from rats artificially infected with, and immunized against, the larval cestode *Cysticercus fasciolaris*. *J. Parasit.*, **42**: 109-121.

207. KRVAVICA, S., MARTINČÍC, T. and ASAJ, R. 1959a. [Metabolism of amino

acids in some parasites. I. Absorption and excretion of amino acids in the tapeworm *Anoplocephala magna*.] *Vet. Arh.*, **29**: 305-313.

208. — 1959b. [Metabolism of amino acids in some parasites. II. Amino acids in the hydatid fluid and germinal layer of *Echinococcus*.] *Vet. Arh.*, **29**: 314-321.

209. LARSH, J. E. 1942. Transmission from mother to offspring of immunity against the mouse cestode *Hymenolepis nana* var. *fraterna*. *Amer. J. Hyg.*, **36**: 187-194.

210. — 1944. Studies on the artificial immunization of mice against infection with the dwarf tapeworm, *Hymenolepis nana* var. *fraterna*. *Amer. J. Hyg.*, **39**: 129-132.

211. — 1951. Host-parasite relationships in cestode infections, with emphasis on host resistance. *J. Parasit.*, **37**: 343-352.

212. LARSH, J. E., RACE, G. J. and ESCH, G. W. 1965. A histopathologic study of mice infected with the larval stage of *Multiceps serialis*. *J. Parasit.*, **51**: 45-52.

213. LAURIE, J. S. 1957. The *in vitro* fermentation of carbohydrates by two species of cestodes and one species of acanthocephala. *Expl Parasit.*, **6**: 245-260.

214. — 1961. Carbohydrate absorption in cestodes from elasmobranch fishes. *Comp. Biochem. Physiol.*, **4**: 63-71.

215. LAWS, G. F. 1968. Physical factors influencing survival of taeniid eggs. *Expl Parasit.*, **22**: 227-239.

215a. LEE, D. L. 1965. *The Physiology of Nematodes*. Oliver & Boyd, Edinburgh and London.

216. — 1966. The structure and composition of the helminth cuticle. *Adv. Parasit.*, **4**: 187-254.

217. LEE, D. L., ROTHMAN, A. H. and SENTURIA, J. B. 1963. Esterases in *Hymenolepis* and in *Hydatigera*. *Expl Parasit.*, **14**: 285-295.

218. LEE, D. L. and TATCHELL, R. J. 1964. Studies on the tapeworm *Anoplocephala perfoliata* (Goeze, 1782). *Parasitology*, **54**: 467-479.

219. LEFEVERE, S. 1952. Sur la phosphatase alcaline chez les cestodes. *Bull. Inst. r. Sci. nat. Belg.*, **28**: 1-4.

220. LEY, J. DE and VERCRUYSSE, R. 1955. Glucose-6-phosphate and gluconate-6-phosphate dehydrogenase in worms. *Biochim. biophys. Acta*, **16**: 615-616.

221. LITCHFORD, R. G. 1963. Observations on *Hymenolepis microstoma* in three laboratory hosts: *Mesocricetus auratus*, *Mus musculus* and *Rattus norvegicus*. *J. Parasit.*, **49**: 403-410.

222. LÖSER, E. 1965a. Der Feinbau des Oogenotop bei cestoden. *Z. ParasitKde*, **25**: 413-458.

223. — 1965b. Die Eibildung bei cestoden. *Z. ParasitKde*, **25**: 556-580.

224. — 1965c. Die postembryonale Entwicklung des Oogenotop bei cestoden. *Z. ParasitKde*, **25**: 581-596.

225. LUKASHENKO, N. P. 1964. [Study of the development of *Alveococcus multilocularis* (Leuckart, 1863) *in vitro*.] In Russian. *Medskaya Parasit.*, **33**: 271-278.

226. LUMSDEN, R. D. 1965. Macromolecular structure of glycogen in some cyclophyllidean and trypanorhynch cestodes. *J. Parasit.*, **51**: 501-515.

227. — 1966a. Cytological studies on the absorptive surfaces of cestodes. I. The fine structure of the strobilar integument. *Z. ParasitKde*, **27**: 355-382.

228. — 1966b. Fine structure of the medullary parenchymal cells of a trypanorhynch cestode, *Lacistorhynchus tenuis* (v. Beneden, 1858), with emphasis on specialisations for glycogen metabolism. *J. Parasit.*, **52**: 417-427.

229. — 1966c. Cytological studies on the absorptive surfaces of cestodes. II. The synthesis and intracellular transport of protein in the strobilar integument of *Hymenolepis diminuta*. *Z. ParasitKde*, **28**: 1-13.

230. — 1967. Ultrastructure of mitochondria in a cestode, *Lacistorhynchus tenuis* (v. Beneden, 1858). *J. Parasit.*, **53**: 65-77.

231. LUMSDEN, R. D. and BYRAM, J. 1967. The ultrastructure of cestode muscle. *J. Parasit.*, **53**: 326-342.

231a. LUMSDEN, R. D. and HARRINGTON, G. W. 1966. Incorporation of linoleic acid by the cestode *Hymenolepis diminuta* (Rudolphi 1819). *J. Parasit.*, **52**: 695-700.

232. McCAIG, M. L. O. and HOPKINS, C. A. 1963. Studies on *Schistocephalus solidus*. II. Establishment and longevity in the definitive host. *Expl Parasit.*, **13**: 273-283.

233. — 1965. Studies on *Schistocephalus solidus*. III. The *in vitro* cultivation of the plerocercoid. *Parasitology*, **55**: 257-268.

234. MACHNICKA-ROGUSKA, B. 1961. Warunki hodowli tasiemcow z rsedu Pseudophyllidea *in vitro*. *Wiad. parazyt.*, **7**: 561-566.

235. — 1965. Preparation of *Taenia saginata* antigens and chemical analysis of antigenic fractions. *Acta parasit. pol.*, **13**: 337-347.

236. MACINNIS, A. J., FISHER, F. M. and READ, C. P. 1965. Membrane transport of purines and pyrimidines in a cestode. *J. Parasit.*, **51**: 260-267.

237. McMAHON, P. A. 1961. Phospholipids of larval and adult *Taenia taeniaeformis*. *Expl Parasit.*, **11**: 156-160.

238. MARKOV, G. S. 1939. Nutrition of tapeworms in artificial media. *Dokl. Akad. Nauk. SSSR.*, **25**: 93-96.

239. MARZULLO, F., SQUADRINI, F. and TAPARELLI, F. 1957. Studio isto-chimico sui parassiti patogeni per l'uomo. Nota II. *Hymenolepis nana, Taenia saginata, Taenia echinococcus. Boll. Soc. med. -chir. Modena*, **57**: 327-331.

240. METTRICK, D. F. and MUNRO, H. N. 1965. Studies on the protein metabolism of cestodes. I. Effect of host dietary constituents on the growth of *Hymenolepis diminuta*. *Parasitology*, **55**: 453-366.

241. MEYER, M. C. and VIK, R. 1963. The life cycle of *Diphyllobothrium sebago* (Ward, 1910). *J. Parasit.*, **49**: 962-968.

242. MEYMARIAN, E. 1961. Host-parasite relationships in echinococcosis. VI. Hatching and activation of *Echinococcus granulosus* ova *in vitro*. *Am. J. trop. Med. Hyg.*, **10**: 719-726.

243. MILLEMANN, R. E.   1955.   Studies on the life-history and biology of *Oochoristica deserti* n. sp. (Cestoda: Linstowiidae) from desert rodents. *J. Parasit.*, **41**: 424-440.

244. MILLER, H. M.   1931.   Immunity of the albino rat to superinfestation with *Cysticercus fasciolaris*. *J. prevent. Med. Baltimore*, **5**: 453-464.

245. MILLER, H. M. and GARDINER, L.   1934.   Further studies on passive immunity to a metazoan parasite, *Cysticercus fasciolaris*. *Am. J. Hyg.*, **20**: 424-431.

246. MILLER, H. M. and MASSIE, E.   1932.   Persistence of acquired immunity to *Cysticercus fasciolaris* after removal of the worms. *J. prev. Med. Baltimore*, **6**: 31-36.

247. MORSETH, D. J.   1965a.   The ultrastructure of taeniid tapeworms. Ph.D. Thesis, University of Dunedin, N.Z.

248. — 1965b.   Ultrastructure of developing taeniid embryophores and associated structures. *Expl Parasit.*, **16**: 207-216.

249. — 1966a.   Chemical composition of embryonic blocks of *Taenia hydatigena*, *Taenia ovis* and *Taenia pisiformis* eggs. *Expl Parasit.*, **18**: 347-354.

250. — 1966b.   The fine structure of the tegument of adult *Echinococcus granulosus*, *Taenia hydatigena* and *Taenia pisiformis*. *J. Parasit.*, **52**: 1074-1085.

251. — 1967a.   The fine structure of the hydatid cyst and the protoscolex of *Echinococcus granulosus*. *J. Parasit.*, **53**: 312-325.

252. — 1967b.   Observations on the fine structure of the nervous system of *Echinococcus granulosus*. *J. Parasit.*, **53**: 492-500.

253. MUELLER, J. F.   1959a.   The laboratory propagation of *Spirometra mansonoides* as an experimental tool. I. Collecting, incubation and hatching of the eggs. *J. Parasit.*, **45**: 353-361.

254. — 1959b.   The laboratory propagation of *Spirometra mansonoides* (Mueller, 1935) as an experimental tool. II. Culture and infection of the copepod host, and harvesting the procercoid. *Trans. Am. microsc. Soc.*, **78**: 245-255.

255. — 1959c.   The laboratory propagation of *Spirometra mansonoides* (Mueller, 1935) as an experimental tool. III. *In vitro* cultivation of the plerocercoid larva in a cell-free medium. *J. Parasit.*, **45**: 561-573.

256. — 1960.   The immunology basis of host specificity in the sparganum larva of *Spirometra mansonoides*. Libro homenaje al Dr. Edvardo Caballero y Caballero. Jubileo 1930-1960 Sobretire, Mexico. 435-442.

257. — 1961a.   The laboratory propagation of *Spirometra mansonoides* as an experimental tool. IV. Experimental inversion of the primary axis in the developing egg. *Expl Parasit.*, **11**: 311-318.

258. — 1961b.   The laboratory propagation of *Spirometra mansonoides* as an experimental tool. V. Behaviour of the sparganum in and out of the mouse host, and formation of immune precipitates. *J. Parasit.*, **47**: 879-883.

259. — 1963. Parasite-induced weight gain in mice. *Ann. N.Y. Acad. Sci.*, **113**: 217-233.

260. — 1965a. Further studies on parasitic obesity in mice, deer mice, and hamsters. *J. Parasit.*, **51**: 523-531.

261. — 1965b. Food intake and weight gain in mice parasitized with *Spirometra mansonoides*. *J. Parasit.*, **51**: 537-540.

262. — 1966a. Host-parasite relationships as illustrated by the cestode *Spirometra mansonoides*. In *Host-Parasite Relationships*. Ed. J. E. McCauley. Oregon State Univ. Press.

263. — 1966b. The laboratory propagation of *Spirometra mansonoides* (Mueller, 1935) as an experimental tool. VII. Improved techniques and additional notes on the biology of the cestode. *J. Parasit.*, **52**: 437-443.

264. MUKHERJEE, T. M. and WILLIAMS, A. W. 1967. A comparative study of the ultrastructure of microvilli in the epithelium of small and large intestine of mice. *J. Cell Biol.*, **34**: 447-461.

265. NAŠKOV, D. and DIMITROVA, E. 1960. [Upon the immunochemical relativity between *M. expansa* and *M. benedeni*.] In Russian. *Bull. Cent. Helm. Lab.*, **5**: 67-70.

266. NASSET, E. S. 1957. Role of the digestive tract in the utilization of protein and amino acids. *J. Am. Med. Ass.*, **164**: 172-177.

267. NASSET, E. S. and JU, J. S. 1961. Mixture of endogenous and exogenous protein in the alimentary tract. *J. Nutr.*, **74**: 461-465.

268. NORMAN, L. and KAGAN, I. G. 1961. The maintenance of *Echinococcus multilocularis* in gerbils (*Meriones unguiculatus*) by intraperitoneal inoculation. *J. Parasit.*, **47**: 870-874.

269. OGREN, R. E. 1955. Development and morphology of glandular regions in oncospheres of *Hymenolepis nana*. *Proc. Pa Acad. Sci.*, **29**: 258-264.

270. — 1957. Morphology and development of oncospheres of the cestode *Oochoristica symmetrica* Baylis, 1927. *J. Parasit.*, **43**: 505-520.

271. — 1958. The hexacanth embryo of a dilepidid tapeworm. I. The development of hooks and contractile parenchyma. *J. Parasit.*, **44**: 477-483.

272. — 1961. The mature oncosphere of *Hymenolepis diminuta*. *J. Parasit.*, **47**: 197-204.

273. — 1962. Continuity of morphology from oncosphere to early cysticercoid in the development of *Hymenolepis diminuta* (Cestoda: Cyclophyllidea). *Expl Parasit.*, **12**: 1-6.

274. — 1967. The cellular pattern in invasive oncospheres of *Hymenolepis diminuta* as revealed by an enzyme-acetic acid-orcein method. *Trans. Am. microsc. Soc.*, **86**: 250-260.

275. OHBAYASHI, M. 1960. Studies on echinococcosis. X. Histological observations in experimental cases of multilocular echinococcosis. *Jap. J. vet. Res.*, **8**: 134-160.

276. ORIHARA, M. 1962. Studies on *Cysticercus fasciolaris*, especially on difference of susceptibility among uniform strains of the mouse. *Jap. J. vet. Res.*, **10**: 37-56.

277. ORR, T. S. C. 1966. Spawning behaviour of rudd, *Scardinius erythrophthalmus* infested with plerocercoids of *Ligula intestinalis*. *Nature, Lond.*, **212**: 736.

278. ORRELL, S. A., BUEDING, E. and COLUCCI, A. V. 1966. Relationship between sedimentation coefficient distribution and glycogen level in the cestode *Hymenolepis diminuta*. *Comp. Biochem. Physiol.*, **18**: 657-662.

279. PASHCHENKO, L. F. 1961. [Early stages of spermatogenesis in *Taenia-rhynchus saginata* Goeze, 1782.] In Russian. *Problemÿ Parazit.*, **1**: 112-122.

280. PAULUZZI, S., SORICE, F., CASTAGNARI, L. and SERRA, P. 1965. Contributo allo studio delle colture *in vitro* degli scolici di *Echinococcus granulosus*. *Annali Sclavo, Sienna*, **7**: 191-218.

281. PAVLOVSKI, E. N. and GNEZDILOV, V. G. 1949. [The factor of intensity in experimental infection with the broad tapeworm.] In Russian. *Dokl. Akad. Nauk. SSSR*, **6**: 755-758.

282. — 1953. [Intra-specific and inter-specific relationship of the components of the parasite biocoenosis in the intestines of the host.] In Russian. *Zool. Zhur.*, **32**: 165-174.

283. PENCE, D. B. 1967. The fine structure and histochemistry of the infective eggs of *Dipylidium caninum*. *J. Parasit.*, **53**: 1041-1054.

284. PENNOIT-DE-COOMAN, E. and GREMBERGEN, G. VAN. 1942. Vergelijkend Onderzoek van het fermentensysteem bij vrijlende en parasitaire plathelminthen. *Verh. K. vlaam. Acad. Wet.*, **4**: 7-77.

285. PHIFER, K. 1958. Aldolase in the larval form of *Taenia crassiceps*. *Expl Parasit.*, **7**: 269-275.

286. — 1960a. Permeation and membrane transport in animal parasites: the absorption of glucose by *Hymenolepis diminuta*. *J. Parasit.*, **46**: 51-62.

287. — 1960b. Permeation and membrane transport in animal parasites: further observations on the uptake of glucose by *Hymenolepis diminuta*. *J. Parasit.*, **46**: 137-144.

288. — 1960c. Permeation and membrane transport in animal parasites: on the mechanism of glucose uptake by *Hymenolepis diminuta*. *J. Parasit.*, **46**: 145-153.

289. POZZI, G. and PIROSKY, I. 1953. Contribución al estudio de la proteina de la hidátide de *Taenia equinococcus*. Análsis cromatográfico en papel. *Arch. intern. Hidatid.*, **13**: 232.

290. PRESCOTT, L. M. and CAMPBELL, J. W. 1965. Phosphoenolpyruvate carboxylase activity and glycogenesis in the flatworm *Hymenolepis diminuta*. *Comp. Biochem. Physiol.*, **14**: 491-511.

291. PYLKKÖ, O. O. 1956a. Studies of the acetylcholine content and cholinesterase activity of the human pathogenic fish tapeworm (*Diphyllobothrium latum*). *Annls Med. exp. Biol. Fenn.*, **34** [Suppl. 8]: 1-81.

292. — 1956b. Cholinesterase in *Diphyllobothrium latum* and *Taenia saginata*. *Annls Med. exp. Biol. Fenn.*, **34**: 328-334.

293. — RACE, G. J., LARSH, J. E., ESCH, G. W. and MARTIN, J. H. 1965. A study of the larval stage of *Multiceps serialis* by electron microscopy. *J. Parasit.*, **51**: 374-369.

294. RAO, K. H. 1960. The problem of Mehlis' gland in helminths with special reference to *Penetrocephalus ganapatii* (Cestoda: Pseudophyllidea) *Parasitology*, **50**: 349-350.

295. RAUSCH, R. L. and JENTOFT, V. L.   1957.   Studies on the helminth fauna of Alaska. XXXI. Observations on the propagation of the larval *Echinococcus multilocularis* Leukart, 1863, *in vitro*. *J. Parasit.*, **43**: 1-8.

296. READ, C. P.   1950.   The vertebrate small intestine as an environment for parasitic helminths. *Rice Inst. Pamph.*, 37, No. 2, 94 pp.

297. — 1951a.   Studies on the enzymes and intermediate products of carbohydrate degradation in the cestode *Hymenolepis diminuta*. *Expl Parasit.*, 1: 1-18.

298. — 1951b.   The ' crowding effect ' in tapeworm infections. *J. Parasit.*, 37: 174-178.

299. — 1952.   Contributions to cestode enzymology. I. The cytochrome system and succinic dehydrogenase in *Hymenolepis diminuta*. *Expl Parasit.*, 1: 353-362.

300. — 1953.   Contributions to cestode enzymology. II. Some anaerobic dehydrogenases in *Hymenolepis diminuta*. *Expl Parasit.*, 2: 341-347.

301. — 1955.   Intestinal physiology and the host-parasite relationship. In: *Some physiological aspects and consequences of parasitism*. 27-49. Ed. W. H. Cole. Rutgers Univ. Press, N.J.

302. — 1956.   Carbohydrate metabolism of *Hymenolepis diminuta*. *Expl Parasit.*, 5: 325-344.

303. — 1957.   The role of carbohydrates in the biology of cestodes. III. Studies on two species from dogfish. *Expl Parasit.*, 6: 288-293.

304. — 1959.   The role of carbohydrates in the biology of cestodes. VIII. Some conclusions and hypotheses. *Expl Parasit.*, 8: 365-382.

305. — 1961.   The carbohydrate metabolism of worms. In: *Comparative physiology of carbohydrate metabolism in heterothermic animals*. Univ. Wash. Press.

306. — 1966.   Nutrition of intestinal helminths. In: *Biology of Parasites. Ed.* Soulsby, E. J. L.   Academic Press.

307. — 1967.   Carbohydrate metabolism in *Hymenolepis* (Cestoda). *J. Parasit.*, 53: 1023-1029.

308. READ, C. P., DOUGLAS, L. T. and SIMMONS, J. E. JR.   1959.   Urea and osmotic properties from elasmobranchs. *Expl Parasit.*, 8: 58-75.

309. READ, C. P. and PHIFER, K.   1959.   The role of carbohydrates in the biology of cestodes. VII. Interactions between individual tapeworms of the same and different species. *Expl Parasit.*, 8: 46-50.

310. READ, C. P. and ROTHMAN, A. H.   1957a.   The role of carbohydrates in the biology of cestodes. I. The effect of dietary carbohydrate quality on the size of *Hymenolepis diminuta*. *Expl Parasit.*, 6: 1-7.

311. — 1957b.   The role of carbohydrates in the biology of cestodes. II. The effect of starvation on glycogenesis and glucose consumption in *Hymenolepis*. *Expl Parasit.*, 6: 280-287.

312. — 1957c.   The role of carbohydrates in the biology of cestodes. IV. Some effects of host dietary carbohydrate on growth and reproduction of *Hymenolepis*. *Expl Parasit.*, 6: 294-305.

313. — 1958.   The role of carbohydrates in the biology of cestodes. VI. The

carbohydrates metabolized *in vitro* by some cyclophyllidean species. *Expl Parasit.*, **7**: 217-223.

314. READ, C. P., ROTHMAN, A. H. and SIMMONS, J. E. 1963. Studies on membrane transport, with special reference to parasite-host integration. *Ann. N.Y. Acad. Sci.*, **113**: 154-205.

315. READ, C. P., SCHILLER, E. L. and PHIFER, K. 1958. The role of carbohydrates in the biology of cestodes. V. Comparative studies on the effects of host dietary carbohydrate on *Hymenolepis* spp. *Expl Parasit.*, **7**: 198-216.

316. READ, C. P. and SIMMONS, J. E. JR. 1963. Biochemistry and physiology of tapeworms. *Physiol. Rev.*, **43**: 263-305.

317. READ, C. P., SIMMONS, J. E. JR., CAMPBELL, J. W. and ROTHMAN, A. H. 1960. Permeation and membrane transport in parasitism: studies on a tapeworm-elasmobranch symbiosis. *Biol. Bull. mar. biol. Lab.*, Woods Hole, **119**: 120-133.

318. READ, C. P., SIMMONS, J. E. JR. and ROTHMAN, A. H. 1960. Permeation and membrane transport in animal parasites: amino acid permeation into tapeworms from elasmobranchs. *J. Parasit.*, **46**: 33-51.

319. REES, G. 1958. A comparison of the structure of the scolex of *Bothriocephalus scorpii* (Müller, 1766) and *Clestobothrium crassiceps* (Reid, 1819), and the mode of attachment of the scolex to the intestine of the host. *Parasitology*, **48**: 468-492.

320. — 1961. Studies on the functional morphology of the scolex and of the genitalia in *Echinobothrium brachysoma* Pintner and *E. affine* Diesing from *Raja clavata* L. *Parasitology*, **51**: 193-226.

321. — 1966. Nerve cells in *Acanthobothrium coronatum* (Rud.) (Cestoda: Tetraphyllidea). *Parasitology*, **56**: 45-54.

322. — 1967. Pathogenesis of adult cestodes. *Helm. Abs.*, **36**: 1-23.

323. REES, G. and WILLIAMS, H. H. 1965. The functional morphology of the scolex and the genitalia of *Acanthobothrium coronatum*. *Parasitology*, **55**: 617-651.

324. REID, W. M. 1942. Certain nutritional requirements of the fowl cestode *Raillietina cesticillus* (Molin) as demonstrated by short periods of starvation of the host. *J. Parasit.*, **28**: 319-340.

325. — 1948. Penetration glands in cyclophyllidean oncospheres. *Trans. Am. microsc. Soc.*, **67**: 177-182.

326. REID, W. M., NICE, S. J. and McINTYRE, R. C. 1949. Certain factors which influence activation of the hexacanth embryo of the fowl tapeworm *Raillietina cesticillus*. *Trans. Ill. St. Acad. Sci.*, **42**: 165-168.

327. RENDTORFF, R. C. 1948. Investigations on the life cycle of *Oöchoristica ratti*, a cestode from rats and mice. *J. Parasit.*, **34**: 243-252.

328. RIGBY, D. W. and MARX, R. A. 1962. A comparative histochemical study of the monogenetic trematode *Rajonchocotyle batis* Cerfontaine with the trypanorhynch cestode *Gilquinia squali* (Fabricius). *Walla Walla Coll. Publs Dep. biol. Sci.*, No. 31: 1-11.

329. ROBERTS, L. S. 1961. The influence of population density on patterns

and physiology of growth in *Hymenolepis diminuta* (Cestoda: Cyclophyllidea) in the definitive host. *Expl Parasit.*, **11**: 332-371.

330. ROBINSON, D. L. H., SILVERMAN, P. H. and PEARCE, A. R. 1963. The culture of *Taenia crassiceps in vitro*. *Trans. R. Soc. trop. Med. Hyg.*, **57**: 238.

331. ROGERS, W. A. and ULMER, M. J. 1962. Effects of continued selfing on *Hymenolepis nana* (Cestoda). *Proc. Iowa Acad. Sci.*, **69**: 557-571.

332. ROGERS, W. P. 1947. Histological distribution of alkaline phosphatase in helminth parasites. *Nature, Lond.*, **159**: 374-375.

333. — 1949. On the relative importance of aerobic metabolism in small nematode parasites of the alimentary canal. I. Oxygen tensions in the normal environment of the parasites. *Austral. J. Sci. Res.*, **2B**: 157-165.

334. — 1962. *The Nature of Parasitism*. Academic Press, London.

335. ROSARIO, B. 1962. The ultrastructure of the cuticle in the cestodes *H. nana* and *H. diminuta*. In: *5th Int. Cong. Electron Microscop.* Ed. S. Bresse. 11-12, Academic Press.

336. — 1964. An electron microscope study of spermatogenesis in cestodes. *J. Ultrastruct. Res.*, **11**: 412-427.

337. ROTHMAN, A. H. 1959a. The physiology of tapeworms, correlated to structures seen with the electron microscope. *J. Parasit.*, **45** (Suppl.): 28.

338. — 1959b. The role of bile salts in the biology of tapeworms. II. Further observations on the effects of bile salts on metabolism. *J. Parasit.*, **45**: 379-383.

339. — 1959c. Studies on the excystment of tapeworms. *Expl Parasit.*, **8**: 336-364.

340. — 1960. Ultramicroscopic evidence of absorptive function in cestodes. *J. Parasit.*, **46** (Suppl.): 10.

341. — 1963. Electron microscopic studies of tapeworms: the surface structures of *Hymenolepis diminuta* (Rudolphi, 1819) Blanchard, 1891. *Trans. Am. microsc. Soc.*, **82**: 22-30.

342. — 1966. Ultrastructural studies of enzyme activity in the cestode cuticle. *Expl Parasit.*, **19**: 332-338.

343. ROTHMAN, A. H. and LEE, D. L. 1963. Histochemical demonstration of dehydrogenase activity in the cuticle of cestodes. *Expl Parasit.*, **14**: 333-336.

344. RUSAK, L. V. 1964a. [Motor reactions of *Hymenolepis nana in vitro*.] In Russian. *Medskaya Parazit.*, **33**: 308-315.

345. — 1964b. [Effect of a number of pharmacological substances on motor reactions of cestodes *in vitro*.] In Russian. *Medskaya Parazit.*, **33**: 582-586.

346. RYBICKA, K. 1957. [On the development of the larvae of the tapeworm *Diorchis ransomi* Schultz, 1940 (*Hymenolepididae*) in the intermediate host.] In Polish. N.S.F. Translation No. OTS 21514. *Acta parasit. pol.*, **5**: 613-644.

347. — 1962a. Observations sur la spermatogenèse d'un cestode Pseudophyllidien, *Triaenophorus lucii* (Müll., 1776). *Ext. Bull. Soc. neuchâtel Sci. nat.*, **85**: 177-181.

348. — 1962b.   La spermatogenèse du cestode *Dipylidium caninum* (L).   *Bull. Soc. zool. Fr.*, **87**: 225-228.

349. — 1964.   Gametogenesis and embryonic development in *Dipylidium caninum*.   *Expl Parasit.*, **15**: 293-313.

350. — 1966.   Embryogenesis in Cestodes.   *Adv. Parasit.*, **4**: 107-186.

351. — 1967.   Embryogenesis in *Hymenolepis diminuta*.   II. Glycogen distribution in the embryos.   *Expl Parasit.*, **20**: 98-105.

352. RYCKE, P. H. DE.   1966.   Development of the cestode *Hymenolepis microstoma* in *Mus musculus*.   *Z. ParasitKde*, **27**: 350-354.

352a. RYCKE, P. H. DE and BERNTZEN, A. K.   1967.   Maintenance and growth of *Hymenolepis microstoma* (Cestoda: Cyclophyllidea) *in vitro*.   *J. Parasit.*, **53**: 352-354.

353. RYCKE, P. H. DE and GREMBERGEN, G. VAN.   1965.   Étude sur l'évagination de scolex d'*Echinococcus granulosus*.   *Z. ParasitKde*, **25**: 518-525.

353a. — 1966.   Study on the evagination of *Cysticercus pisiformis*.   *Z. ParasitKde*, **27**: 341-349.

354. SADUN, E. H., WILLIAMS, J. S., MERONEY, F. C. and MUELLER, J. F.   1965.   Biochemical changes in mice infected with spargana of the cestode *Spirometra mansonoides*.   *J. Parasit.*, **51**: 532-536.

355. SALT, G.   1963.   The defence reactions of insects to metazoan parasites.   *Parasitology*, **53**: 527-642.

356. SAWADA, I.   1953.   On the life history of the poultry cestode, *Raillietina (Raillietina) echinobothrida*.   *Zool. Mag., Tokyo*, **62**: 202-205.

357. — 1959a.   Experimental studies on the evagination of the cysticercoids of *Raillietina kashiwarensis*.   *Expl Parasit.*, **8**: 325-335.

358. — 1959b.   Studies on the life history of the chicken tapeworm, *Raillietina (Paroniella) kashiwarensis* Sawada.   *J. Nara Gakugei Univ.*, **8**: 31-63.

359. — 1960a.   Studies on the artificial hatching of oncospheres of the fowl tapeworm, *Raillietina cesticillus*.   *Zool. Mag., Tokyo*, **69**: 142-149.

360. — 1960b.   Penetration glands in onchospheres of the chicken tapeworms, *Raillietina echinobothrida* and *Raillietina kashiwarensis*.   *Z. ParasitKde*, **20**: 350-354.

361. — 1961.   Penetration glands in the onchospheres of *Raillietina cesticillus*.   *Expl Parasit.*, **11**: 141-146.

362. — 1967.   Artificial hatching of the fowl tapeworm *Raillietina echinobothrida* onchosphere.   *Bull. Nara Univ. Ed.*, **15**: 27-35.

363. SCHARDEIN, J. L. and WAITZ, J. A.   1955.   Histochemical studies of esterases in the cuticle and nerve cords of four cyclophyllidean cestodes.   *J. Parasit.*, **51**: 356-363.

364. SCHEIBEL, L. W. and SAZ, H. J.   1966.   The pathway for anaerobic carbohydrate dissimilation in *Hymenolepis diminuta*.   *Comp. Biochem. Physiol.*, **18**: 151-162.

365. SCHILLER, E. L.   1955.   Studies on the helminth fauna of Alaska.   XXVI.   Some observations on the cold-resistance of eggs of *Echinococcus sibiricensis* Rausch & Schiller, 1954.   *J. Parasit.*, **41**: 578-582.

366. — 1959a.   Experimental studies on morphological variation in the cestode

genus *Hymenolepis*. I. Morphology and development of the cystercoid of *H. nana* in *Tribolium confusum*. *Expl Parasit.*, **8**: 91-118.

367. — 1959b. Experimental studies on morphological variation in the cestode genus *Hymenolepis*. II. Growth, development and reproduction of the strobilate phase of *H. nana* in different mammalian host species. *Expl Parasit.*, **8**: 215-235.

368. — 1959c. Experimental studies on morphological variation in the cestode genus *Hymenolepis*. III. X-Irradiation as a mechanism for facilitating analyses in *H. nana*. *Expl Parasit.*, **8**: 427-470.

369. — 1959d. Experimental studies on morphological variation in the cestode genus *Hymenolepis*. IV. Influence of the host on variation in *H. nana*. *Expl Parasit.*, **8**: 581-590.

370. — 1965. A simplified method for the *in vitro* cultivation of the rat tapeworm *Hymenolepis diminuta*. *J. Parasit.*, **51**: 516-518.

371. SCHILLER, E. L., READ, C. P. and ROTHMAN, A. H. 1959. Preliminary experiments on the growth of a cyclophyllidean cestode *in vitro*. *J. Parasit.*, **45**: (Suppl.): 29.

372. SCHWABE, C. W. 1955. Helminth parasites and neoplasia. *Am. J. vet. Res.*, **16**: 485-488.

373. — 1959. Host-parasite relationships in Echinococcosis. I. Observations on the permeability of the hydatid cyst wall. *Amer. J. trop. Med. Hyg.*, **8**: 20-28.

374. SCHWABE, C. W., KOUSSA, M. and ACRA, A. N. 1961. Host-parasite relationships in echinococcosis. IV. Acetylcholinesterase and permeability regulation in the hydatid cyst wall. *Comp. Biochem. Physiol.*, **2**: 161-172.

375. SCOTT, D. B., NYLEN, M. U., BRAND, T. VON, and PUGH, M. H., 1962. The mineralogical composition of the calcareous corpuscles of *Taenia taeniaeformis*. *Expl Parasit.*, **12**: 445-458.

376. SCOTT, J. S. 1965a. The development and morphology of *Polycercus lumbrici* (Cestoda: Cyclophyllidea). *Parasitology*, **55**: 127-143.

377. — 1965b. Evagination of the cysticercoid in *Polycercus lumbrici*. *Parasitology*, **55**: 421-425.

378. SENTURIA, J. B. 1964. Studies on the absorption of methionine by the cestode, *Hymenolepis citelli*. *Comp. Biochem. Physiol.*, **12**: 259-272.

379. SHEEHY, T. W. and FLOCH, M. H. 1964. *The small intestine: its functions and diseases*. Hoeber Medical Division, Harper & Row.

380. SHIELD, J. 1969. Histochemical studies on cholinesterases of the cyclophyllidean cestodes *Dipylidium caninum*, *Echinococcus granulosus* and *Hydatigera taeniaeformis*. *Expl Parasit.* (In press.)

381. SHIKHOBALOVA, N. P. 1950. [Questions of immunity in helminthiasis.] U.S. translation available. *Acad. Sci. USSR Publications*, Moscow.

382. SHORB, D. A. 1933. Host-parasite relations of *Hymenolepis fraterna* in the rat and the mouse. *Amer. J. Hyg.*, **18**: 74-113.

383. SHULTS, R. S. and ISMAGILOVA, R. G. 1962. [On new immunological reactions in Echinococcosis.] In Russian. *Vest. sel'. -khoz. Nauki, Alma-Ata*, **5**: 45-49.

248 THE PHYSIOLOGY OF CESTODES

384. SIDDIQI, A. H. 1961a. Studies on the morphology of *Cotugnia digonopora* Pasquale 1890 (Cestoda: Davaineidae). Part IV. Excretory system. *Z. ParasitKde*, **21**: 93-100.

385. — 1961b. Studies on the morphology of *Cotugnia digonopora* Pasquale 1890 (Cestoda: Davaineidae). Part V. Nervous system. *Z. ParasitKde*. **21**: 101-112.

386. SILVERMAN, P. H. 1954a. Studies on the biology of some tapeworms of the genus *Taenia*. I. Factors affecting hatching and activation of taeniid ova, and some criteria of their viability. *Ann. trop. Med. Parasit.*, **48**: 207-215.

387. — 1954b. Studies on the biology of some tapeworms of the genus *Taenia*. II. The morphology and development of the taeniid hexacanth embryo and its enclosing membranes, with some notes on the state of development and propagation of gravid segments. *Ann. trop. Med. Parasit.*, **48**: 355-366.

388. — 1955. A technique for studying the *in vitro* effect of serum on activated taeniid hexacanth embryos. *Nature, Lond.*, **176**: 598-599.

389. — 1965. *In vitro* cultivation procedures for parasitic helminths. *Adv. Parasit.*, **3**: 159-222.

390. SILVERMAN, P. H. and MANEELY, R. B. 1955. Studies on the biology of some tapeworms of the genus *Taenia*. III. The role of the secreting gland of the hexacanth embryo in the penetration of the intestinal mucosa of the intermediate host, and some of its histochemical reactions. *Ann. trop. Med. Parasit.*, **49**: 326-330.

391. SIMMONS, J. E. JR. 1961. Urease activity in trypanorhynch cestodes. *Biol. Bull. mar. biol. lab., Woods Hole*, **121**: 535-546.

392. SINGH, K. S. and SINGH, K. P. 1958. Morphology and histochemistry of interproglottidal glands of *Moniezia expansa*. *Indian J. Helminth.*, **10**: 111-131.

393. SINHA, D. P. and HOPKINS, C. A. 1967a. *In vitro* cultivation of the tapeworm *Hymenolepis nana* from larva to adult. *Nature, Lond.*, **215**: 1275-1276.

394. — 1967b. Studies on *Schistocephalus solidus*. IV. The effect of temperature on growth and maturation *in vitro*. *Parasitology*, **57**: 555-566.

395. SJÖSTRAND, F. S. 1967. The structure of cellular membranes. *Protoplasma*, **63**: 248-261.

396. SKWORZOV, A. A. 1942-3. Egg structure of *Taeniarhynchus saginatus* and its control. *Zool. Zh.*, **21/22**: 15-18.

397. ŠLAIS, J. 1958. Tasemnice *Davainea proglottina* u. slepic. Příspevěk k mechanismu přichyeři a změn ve střevní sliznici. *Ceskosl. Biol.*, **7**: 456-461.

398. — 1961. Damage of the intestinal mucous membrane by tapeworms *Aploparaxis furcigera* (Rudolphi) and *Hymenolepis parvula* (Kowalewski) in ducks. *Helminthologia*, **3**: 316-321.

399. — 1964. Histologic studies in cysticercosis of the brain. *Wiad. parazyt.*, **10**: 313-314.

400. 1966a. Die Analogie der Morphologie und Entwicklung zwischen dem

Trophoblast und dem Bläschen der Cysticercuslarven der Bandwürmer. *Anat. Anz.*, **118**: 495-502.

401. — 1966b. Beitrag zur Morphogenese des *Cysticercus cellulosae* und *C. bovis*. *Folia parasit.* (*Praha*), **13**: 73-92.

402. — 1966c. The importance of the bladder for the development of the cysticercus. *Parasitology*, **56**: 707-713.

402a. SMITH, H. and SMYTH, J. D. 1968. Unpublished work.

403. SMYTH, D. H. 1963. Intestinal absorption. In: *Recent Advances in Physiology*. (8th edition). Churchill, London.

404. SMYTH, D. H. (Ed.) 1967. *Intestinal Absorption*. *Br. med. Bull.*, **23**: 205-290.

405. SMYTH, J. D. 1946. Studies on tapeworm physiology. I. The cultivation of *Schistocephalus solidus in vitro*. *J. exp. Biol.*, **23**: 47-70.

406. — 1947a. The physiology of tapeworms. *Biol. Rev.*, **22**: 214-238.

407. — 1947b. Studies on tapeworm physiology. II. Cultivation and development of *Ligula intestinalis in vitro*. *Parasitology*, **38**: 173-181.

408. — 1950. Studies on tapeworm physiology. V. Further observations on the maturation of *Schistocephalus solidus* (Diphyllobothriidae) under sterile conditions *in vitro*. *J. Parasit.*, **36**: 371-383.

409. — 1952. Studies on tapeworm physiology. VI. Effect of temperature on the maturation *in vitro* of *Schistocephalus solidus*. *J. exp. Biol.*, **29**: 304-309.

410. — 1954a. Studies on tapeworm physiology. VII. Fertilization of *Schistocephalus solidus in vitro*. *Expl Parasit.*, **3**: 64-71.

411. — 1954b. A technique for the histochemical demonstration of polyphenol oxidase and its application to egg-shell formation in helminths and byssus formation in *Mytilus*. *Q. Jl. microsc. Sci.*, **95**: 139-152.

412. — 1955. Problems relating to the *in vitro* cultivation of pseudophyllidean cestodes from egg to adult. *Rev. Iber. Parasit.*, Tomo Extraordinario, 65-86.

413. — 1956. Studies on tapeworm physiology. IX. Histochemical study of egg-shell formation in *Schistocephalus solidus* (Pseudophyllidea). *Expl Parasit.*, **5**: 519-540.

414. — 1958. Cultivation and development of larval cestode fragments *in vitro*. *Nature, Lond.*, **181**: 1119-1122.

415. — 1959. Maturation of larval pseudophyllidean cestodes and strigeid trematodes under axenic conditions; the significance of nutritional levels in platyhelminth development. *Ann. N.Y. Acad. Sci.*, **77**: 102-125.

416. — 1962a. Lysis of *Echinococcus granulosus* by surface-active agents in bile and the role of this phenomenon in determining host specificity in helminths. *Proc. Roy. Soc., B*, **156**: 553-572.

417. — 1962b. *Introduction to Animal Parasitology*. English Universities Press, London.

418. — 1962c. Studies on tapeworm physiology. X. Axenic cultivation of the hydatid organism, *Echinococcus granulosus*; establishment of a basic technique. *Parasitology*, **52**: 441-457.

419. — 1963. Biology of cestode life-cycles. *Comm. Agric. Bureau*, No. 34, 1-38.

420. — 1964a. Observations on the scolex of *Echinococcus granulosus*, with special reference to the occurrence and cytochemistry of secretory cells in the rostellum. *Parasitology*, **54**: 515-526.

421. — 1964b. The biology of the hydatid organisms. *Adv. Parasit.*, **2**: 169-219.

422. — 1966. *The Physiology of Trematodes*. Oliver & Boyd, Edinburgh and London.

423. — 1967. Studies on tapeworm physiology. XI. *In vitro* cultivation of *Echinococcus granulosus* from the protoscolex to the strobilate stage. *Parasitology*, **57**: 111-133.

423a. — 1969. Parasites as biological models. *Parasitology*, **59**: 73-91.

424. SMYTH, J. D. and CLEGG, J. A. 1959. Egg-shell formation in trematodes and cestodes. *Expl Parasit.*, **8**: 286-323.

425. SMYTH, J. D., GEMMELL, M. A. and SMYTH, M. M. 1969. The establishment of *Echinococcus granulosus* in the intestine of normal and vaccinated dogs. *Indian J. Helminth. Srivastava Commemoration Volume*.

426. SMYTH, J. D. and HASLEWOOD, G. A. D. 1963. The biochemistry of bile as a factor in determining host specificity in intestinal parasites, with particular reference to *Echinococcus granulosus*. *Ann. N.Y. Acad. Sci.*, **113**: 234-260.

427. SMYTH, J. D. and HOWKINS, A. B. 1966. An *in vitro* technique for the production of eggs of *Echinococcus granulosus* by maturation of partly developed strobila. *Parasitology*, **56**: 763-766.

428. SMYTH, J. D., HOWKINS, A. B. and BARTON, M. 1966. Factors controlling the differentiation of the hydatid organism, *Echinococcus granulosus* into cystic or strobilar stages *in vitro*. *Nature, Lond.*, **211**: 1374-1377.

429. SMYTH, J. D. and MILLER, H. J. 1968. Unpublished work.

430. SMYTH, J. D., MILLER, H. J. and HOWKINS, A. B. 1967. Further analysis of the factors controlling strobilization, differentiation and maturation of *Echinococcus granulosus in vitro*. *Expl Parasit.*, **21**: 31-41.

431. SMYTH, J. D., MORGAN, J., MORGAN, W. T. J. and WATKINS, W. M. 1966. Unpublished work.

432. SMYTH, J. D., MORSETH, D. J. and SMYTH, M. M. 1968. Observations on nuclear secretions in the rosteller gland cells of *Echinococcus granulosus* (Cestoda). *The Nucleus*. (In press.)

433. SMYTH, J. D. and SMYTH, M. M. 1964. Natural and experimental hosts of *Echinococcus granulosus* and *E. multilocularis*, with comments on the genetics of speciation in the genus *Echinococcus*. *Parasitology*, **54**: 493-514.

434. — 1968. Some aspects of host specificity in the *Echinococcus granulosus*. *Helminthologia*, **9**: 519-529.

435. SOULSBY, E. J. L. 1962. Antigen-antibody reactions in helminth infections. *Adv. Immun.*, **2**: 265-308.

436. — 1962b. Immunity to helminths and its effect on helminth infections.

In: Animal Health and Production. (Eds. Grunsell, C. S.; Wright, A. I.). Butterworths, London.

437. — 1963. Immunological unresponsiveness to helminth infections in animals. *Proc. 17th World Vet. Congr., 1963,* 1: 761-767.

438. — (Ed.) 1966. *Biology of Parasites.* Academic Press, New York.

439. SPECHT, D. and VOGE, M. 1965. Asexual multiplication of *Mesocestoides* tetrathyridia in laboratory animals. *J. Parasit.,* 51: 268-272.

440. SPECTOR, W. G. 1964. The acute inflammatory response (Conference on:). *Ann. N.Y. Acad., Sci.,* 116: (Art 3) 747-1084.

441. SPRENT, J. F. A. 1963. *Parasitism.* University of Queensland Press, Brisbane.

442. SUTER, E. and RAMSEIER, H. 1964. Cellular reactions in infection. *Adv. Immun.,* 4: 117-173.

443. SWEATMAN, G. K. 1957. Acquired immunity in lambs infected with *Taenia hydatigena* Pallas, 1766. *Canad. J. comp. Med.,* 21: 65-71.

444. SWEATMAN, G. K., WILLIAMS, R. J., MORIARTY, K. M. and HENSHALL, T. C. 1963. On acquired immunity to *Echinococcus granulosus* in sheep. *Res. vet. Sci.,* 4: 187-198.

445. TAKAHASHI, T. 1959a. [Studies on *Diphyllobothrium mansoni.* I. Life cycle and host specificity.] (In Japanese; English summary.) *Jap. J. Parasit.,* 8: 567-574.

446. — 1959b. [Studies on *Diphyllobothrium mansoni.* II. Histochemical studies on plerocercoid.] (In Japanese; English summary) *Jap. J. Parasit.,* 10: 669-676.

447. TAN, B. D. and JONES, A. W. 1966. X-ray induced abnormalities and recovery in *Hymenolepis microstoma. Expl Parasit.,* 18: 355-373.

448. TAYLOR, A. E. R. 1961. Axenic culture of the rodent tapeworms *Hymenolepis diminuta* and *H. nana. Expl Parasit.,* 11: 176-187.

449. — 1963. Maintenance of larval *Taenia crassiceps* (Cestoda: Cyclophyllidea) in a chemically defined medium. *Expl Parasit.,* 14: 304-310.

450. TAYLOR, A. E. R. and BAKER, J. R. 1968. *Cultivation of Parasites* in vitro. Oxford: Blackwell Sci. Publ.

451. TAYLOR, A. E. R. and HAYNES, W. D. G. 1966. Studies on the metabolism of larval tapeworms (Cyclophyllidea: *Taenia crassiceps*). I. Amino acid composition before and after *in vitro* culture. *Expl Parasit.,* 18: 327-331.

452. TAYLOR, A. E. R., McCABE, M. and LONGMUIR, I. S. 1966. Studies on the metabolism of larval tapeworms (Cyclophyllidea: *Taenia crassiceps*). II. Respiration, glycogen utilization, and lactic acid production during culture in a chemically defined medium. *Expl Parasit.,* 19: 269-275.

453. THOMPSON, M. J., MOSETTIG, E. and BRAND, T. VON, 1960. Unsaponifiable lipids of *Taenia taeniaeformis* and *Moniezia* sp. *Expl Parasit.,* 9: 127-130.

454. THREADGOLD, L. T. 1962. An electron microscope study of the tegument and associated structures of *Dipylidium caninum. Q. Jl. microsc. Sci.,* 103: 135-140.

455. THREADGOLD, L. T. 1964. The ultrastructure of the tegument of *Proteocephalus pollanicoli. 3rd Europ. Reg. Conf. Electron Microscopy*, 563-564.

456. TIMOFEEV, V. A. 1964. [Structure of the cuticle of *Schistocephalus pungitii* in the different phases of its development in connection with the specific feeding habits of the cestodes. Electron and luminescent microscopy of the cell.] (In Russian; English summary.) *Ref. Zh. Biol.*, 1965, No. 16K48, 50-60. Nauka: Moscow and Leningrad.

457. UGOLEV, A. M. 1965. Membrane (contact) digestion. *Physiol. Rev.*, **45**: 555-595.

458. URQUHART, G. M., JARRETT, W. F. H. and MULLIGAN, W. 1962. Helminth immunity. *Adv. vet. Sci.*, **7**: 87-129.

459. VILLELLA, J. B., GOULD, S. E. and GOMBERG, H. J. 1960. Effect of cobalt 60 and X-ray on infectivity of cysticercoids of *Hymenolepis diminuta*. *J. Parasit.*, **46**: 165-169.

460. VOGE, M. 1959. Sensitivity of developing *Hymenolepis diminuta* larvae to high temperature stress. *J. Parasit.*, **45**: 175-181.

461. — 1961a. Effect of high temperature stress on histogenesis in the cysticercoid of *Hymenolepis diminuta* (Cestoda: Cyclophyllidea). *J. Parasit.*, **47**: 189-195.

462. — 1961b. Observations on development and high temperature sensitivity of cysticercoids of *Raillietina cesticillus* and *Hymenolepis citelli* (Cestoda: Cyclophyllidea). *J. Parasit.*, **47**: 839-841.

463. — 1963. Maintenance *in vitro* of *Taenia crassiceps* cysticerci. *J. Parasit.*, **49** (Suppl.): 59-60.

464. — 1967. Development *in vitro* of *Mesocestoides* from oncosphere to young tetrathyridium. *J. Parasit.*, **53**: 78-82.

465. VOGE, M. and BERNTZEN, A. K. 1961. *In vitro* hatching of oncospheres of *Hymenolepis diminuta* (Cestoda: Cyclophyllidea). *J. Parasit.*, **47**: 813-818.

466. VOGE, M. and COULOMBE, L. S. 1966. Growth and asexual multiplication *in vitro* of *Mesocestoides* tetrathyridia. *Am. J. trop. Med. Hyg.*, **15**: 902-907.

467. VOGE, M. and HEYNEMAN, D. 1957. Development of *Hymenolepis nana* and *Hymenolepis diminuta* (Cestoda: Hymenolepidae) in the intermediate host *Tribolium confusum. Univ. Calif. Publs Zool.*, **59**: 549-579.

468. VOGE, M. and TURNER, J. A. 1956. Effect of temperature on larval development of the cestode, *Hymenolepis diminuta. Expl Parasit.*, **5**: 580-586.

469. WAITZ, J. A. 1963. Histochemical studies on the cestode *Hydatigera taeniaeformis. J. Parasit.*, **49**: 73-80.

470. WAITZ, J. A. and SCHARDEIN, J. A. 1964. Histochemical studies of four cyclophyllidean cestodes. *J. Parasit.*, **50**: 271-277.

471. WARDLE, R. A. and McLEOD, J. A. 1952. *The Zoology of Tapeworms*. Minnesota Press.

472. WARREN, McW. and DAUGHERTY, J. 1957. Host effects on the lipid fraction of *Hymenolepis diminuta. J. Parasit.*, **43**: 521-526.

473. WEBSTER, G. A. and CAMERON, T. W. M. 1963. Some preliminary observations on the development of *Echinococcus in vitro*. *Can. J. Zool.*, **41**: 185-194.

474. WEINMANN, C. J. 1964. Host resistance to *Hymenolepis nana*. II. Specificity of resistance to reinfection in the direct cycle. *Expl Parasit.*, **15**: 514-526.

475. — 1966. Immunity mechanisms in cestode infections. In: *Biology of Parasites. Ed.* Soulsby, E. J. L. Academic Press, New York.

476. WEINSTEIN, P. P. 1966. The *in vitro* cultivation of helminths with reference to morphogenesis. In: *Biology of Parasites. Ed.* Souslby, E. J. L. Academic Press, New York.

477. WERTHEIM, G., ZELEDON, R. and READ, C. P. 1960. Transaminases of tapeworms. *J. Parasit.*, **46**: 497-499.

478. W.H.O. 1964. *Immunological Methods*. Blackwell Sci. Pubs., Oxford.

479. W.H.O. 1965. Immunology and parasitic diseases. *W.H.O. Techn. Rep.*, No. 315, 1-64.

480. WIKGREN, B-J. P. 1966. The effect of temperature on the cell division cycle in diphyllobothrid plerocercoids. *Acta zool. Fenn.*, **114**: 3-27.

481. WIKGREN, B-J. P. and NIKANDER, P. 1964. Cause of death of plerocercoids of *Diphyllobothrium latum* (L.) at low temperatures *Memo. Soc. Faun. Flora fenn.*, **40**: 189-192.

482. WILLIAMS, H. H. 1960a. Some observations on *Parabothrium gadipollachii* (Rudolphi, 1810) and *Abothrium gadi* van Beneden 1870 (Cestoda: Pseudophyllidea) including an account of their mode of attachment and of variation in the two species. *Parasitology*, **50**: 303-322.

483. — 1960b. The intestine in members of the genus *Raja* and host-specificity in the Tetraphyllidea. *Nature, Lond.*, **188**: 514-516.

484. — 1961. Observations on *Echeneibothrium maculatum* (Cestoda: Tetraphyllidea). *J. mar. biol. Ass. U.K.*, **41**: 631-652.

485. — 1967. Helminth diseases of fish. *Helm. Abs.*, **36**: 261-295.

486. WILSON, T. H. 1962. *Intestinal Absorption*. W. B. Saunders, London.

487. WISEMAN, G. 1964. *Absorption from the Intestine*. Academic Press, London & New York.

488. YAMAO, Y. 1952a. [Histochemical studies on endoparasites. VII. Distribution of the glycero-mono-phosphatases in the tissues of the cestodes, *Anoplocephala perfoliata*, *A. magna*, *Moniezia benedeni*, *M. expansa* and *Taenia taeniaeformis*.] (In Japanese: English summary.) *Zool. Mag., Tokyo*, **61**: 254-260.

489. — 1952b. [Histochemical studies on endoparasites. VIII. Distribution of the glycero-mono-phosphatases in various tissues of larvae of cestodes, *Cysticercus bovis*, *Echinococcus cysticus fertilis* and *Cysticercus fasciolaris*.] (In Japanese: English summary.) *Zool. Mag., Tokyo*, **61**: 290-294.

490. — 1952c. [Histochemical studies on endoparasites. IX. On the distribution of glycogen.] (In Japanese; English summary.) *Zool. Mag., Tokyo*, **61**: 317-322.

491. YAMASHITA, J. 1960. On the susceptibility and histogenesis of *Echinococcus multilocularis* in the experimental mouse with the state of echinococcosis in Japan. *Parrassitologia*, **2**: 399-406.

492. YAMASHITA, J., OBHAYASHI, M., SAKAMOTO, T. and ORIHARA, M. E. 1962. Studies on echinococcosis. XIII. Observation on the vesicular development of the scolex of *Echinococcus multilocularis in vitro. Jap. J. vet. Res.*, **10**: 85-96.

Index

A number in **heavy type** refers to an illustration on that page.

255